THE COLLAGEN DIET COOKBOOK FOR WOMEN OVER 50

Unlocking Vitality: Harnessing the Power of Collagen for Radiant Health

Ramon Francisco

Copyright © 2024

All Rights Are Reserved

The content in this book may not be reproduced, duplicated, or transferred without the express written permission of the author or publisher. Under no circumstances will the publisher or author be held liable or legally responsible for any losses, expenditures, or damages incurred directly or indirectly as a consequence of the information included in this book.

Legal Remarks

Copyright protection applies to this publication. It is only intended for personal use. No piece of this work may be modified, distributed, sold, quoted, or paraphrased without the author's or publisher's consent.

Disclaimer Statement

Please keep in mind that the contents of this booklet are meant for educational and recreational purposes. Every effort has been made to offer accurate, up-to-date, reliable, and thorough information. There are, however, no stated or implied assurances of any kind. Readers understand that the author is providing competent counsel. The content in this book originates from several sources. Please seek the opinion of a competent professional before using any of the tactics outlined in this book. By reading this book, the reader agrees that the author will not be held accountable for any direct or indirect damages resulting from the use of the information contained therein, including, but not limited to, errors, omissions, or inaccuracies.

Table of Contents

INTRODUCTION

Welcome to "The Collagen Diet Cookbook for Women Over 50"! If you're holding this book in your hands, chances are you're on a quest for radiant health, vitality, and a little extra spring in your step. Well, my friend, you've come to the right place. Let's embark on this journey together, shall we?

But first, let me pull up a chair, pour you a cup of herbal tea (or maybe a glass of collagen-infused lemon water if you're feeling fancy), and let's have a heart-to-heart chat. Picture this: you're in your fifties, navigating the beautiful chaos of life, juggling career, family, and perhaps the occasional existential crisis. Sound familiar? Trust me, I've been there. And let's be real, sometimes it feels like the universe decided to throw in a few extra curveballs just for good measure, right? But fear not, my fellow fabulous fifty-something! You're not alone, and you're stronger and more resilient than you give yourself credit for.

Now, let's address the elephant in the room – aging. Yep, I said it. Aging. It's a word that often comes with a hefty side serving of societal expectations, stereotypes, and downright ridiculous notions about what it means to be a woman over 50. But here's the thing: age is just a number, and its high time we redefine what it means to thrive in our golden years. Enter the collagen diet – your secret weapon for embracing aging with grace, vitality, and a sprinkle of sass. But hold on, before you start picturing yourself sipping kale smoothies while doing yoga on a mountaintop (although if that's your thing, more power to you!), let me assure you – this isn't your typical "diet" book. No calorie counting, no deprivation, and definitely no shame-inducing lectures about your love affair with chocolate (hey, we all have our vices).

Instead, think of this book as your culinary roadmap to nourishing your body from the inside out, with a little sprinkle of collagen magic thrown in for good measure. We're talking about vibrant, delicious meals that not only tantalize your taste buds but also support your body's natural collagen production – the key to plump skin, strong nails, luscious hair, and joints that move with the grace of a gazelle (well, almost).

But wait, I hear you asking, what exactly is collagen, and why should I care? Ah, my dear reader, allow me to enlighten you. Collagen is the most abundant protein in your body, acting as the glue that holds everything together – think of it as the scaffolding that keeps your skin firm, your bones strong, and your joints flexible. In short, collagen is your body's best friend, and its high time we show it some love.

Now, I won't sugarcoat it – getting older isn't always a walk in the park. We're faced with a myriad of challenges – hormonal changes, metabolism slowdowns, and let's not even get started on those pesky gray hairs that seem to pop up overnight (seriously, where do they come from?). But here's the good news – by nourishing your body with collagen-rich foods, you can support your body's natural repair mechanisms, slow down the aging process, and embrace your inner goddess with open arms.

But before we dive headfirst into the delicious recipes awaiting you in these pages, let's take a moment to set the stage for success. In the following chapters, we'll cover everything from stocking your kitchen with collagen-boosting goodies to crafting mouthwatering meals that will have you licking your plate clean (no judgment here, my friend).

So grab your apron, sharpen those knives, and get ready to embark on a culinary adventure like no other. Whether you're a seasoned chef or a kitchen newbie, there's something here for everyone. So here's to you, my fabulous fifty-something – may your collagen be plentiful, your laughter contagious, and your kitchen filled with love and deliciousness. Let's do this!

GETTING STARTED WITH THE COLLAGEN DIET COOKBOOK FOR WOMEN OVER 50

Welcome to the beginning of your journey towards radiant health and vitality with the Collagen Diet Cookbook for Women Over 50. In this chapter, we'll lay the groundwork for your success by helping you assess your collagen needs, stocking your kitchen with essential ingredients, and understanding the basics of the collagen diet. So grab a pen and paper, and let's dive in!

Assessing Your Collagen Needs

Before we delve into the specifics of the collagen diet, it's essential to understand why collagen is crucial for women over 50 and how to assess your individual needs. Collagen is a structural protein found abundantly in your skin, bones, muscles, tendons, and ligaments. As we age, our body's natural collagen production declines, leading to visible signs of aging such as wrinkles, sagging skin, joint pain, and brittle nails.

Assessing your collagen needs begins with understanding your current health status and lifestyle factors that may impact collagen production. Factors such as age, diet, hormonal changes, sun exposure, smoking, and stress can all influence collagen synthesis and degradation.

If you're experiencing any of the following symptoms, it may indicate that your collagen levels are lower than optimal:

- Fine lines and wrinkles
- Sagging skin

- Joint pain or stiffness

- Brittle nails

- Thinning hair

- Slow wound healing

Additionally, certain medical conditions such as osteoarthritis, osteoporosis, and autoimmune disorders can affect collagen metabolism and require special attention.

Once you've identified your potential collagen needs, it's time to consider how the collagen diet can help replenish and support your body's collagen stores.

Stocking Your Kitchen for Success

Now that you're aware of the importance of collagen in maintaining your overall health and vitality, let's turn our attention to stocking your kitchen with the right ingredients to support your collagen journey.

The key to success on the collagen diet is to focus on whole, nutrient-dense foods that are rich in collagen-building nutrients. Here are some essential ingredients to add to your shopping list:

- **Collagen-Rich Foods**: Incorporate foods that are naturally high in collagen or support collagen production, such as bone broth, wild-caught fish, grass-fed beef, pasture-raised poultry, and eggs.

- **Vitamin C-Rich Foods**: Vitamin C is essential for collagen synthesis, so be sure to include plenty of fruits and vegetables such as citrus fruits, strawberries, kiwi, bell peppers, and dark leafy greens in your diet.

- **Antioxidant-Rich Foods**: Antioxidants help protect collagen from damage caused by free radicals, so load up on colorful fruits and vegetables, nuts, seeds, and herbs such as berries, spinach, kale, nuts, seeds, and green tea.

- **Healthy Fats**: Omega-3 fatty acids found in fatty fish, flaxseeds, chia seeds, and walnuts help reduce inflammation and support skin health.

- **Hydrating Beverages**: Stay hydrated with plenty of water, herbal teas, and coconut water, which help maintain skin elasticity and hydration.

- **Herbs and Spices**: Flavor your meals with anti-inflammatory herbs and spices such as turmeric, ginger, cinnamon, and garlic, which support overall health and wellbeing.

By stocking your kitchen with these collagen-boosting ingredients, you'll have everything you need to create delicious and nutritious meals that support your body's collagen production and promote optimal health and vitality.

Understanding the Basics of the Collagen Diet

Now that you've assessed your collagen needs and stocked your kitchen with collagen-boosting ingredients, let's take a closer look at the basics of the collagen diet and how to incorporate it into your lifestyle.

The collagen diet focuses on consuming foods that support collagen production while avoiding those that may deplete collagen levels or hinder absorption. Here are some key principles to keep in mind:

- **Focus on Whole Foods**: Choose whole, unprocessed foods whenever possible, and limit your intake of refined sugars, processed foods, and artificial additives, which can contribute to inflammation and collagen breakdown.

- **Prioritize Protein**: Include adequate protein sources in your diet to provide the building blocks for collagen synthesis. Opt for high-quality protein sources such as lean meats, poultry, fish, eggs, dairy, legumes, and plant-based protein sources such as tofu, tempeh, and lentils.

- **Support Nutrient Absorption**: Certain nutrients are essential for collagen synthesis, so be sure to consume a varied diet rich in vitamins, minerals, and antioxidants. In addition to vitamin C, other nutrients that support collagen production include vitamin E, zinc, copper, and sulfur.

- **Stay Hydrated**: Adequate hydration is essential for maintaining skin elasticity and hydration. Aim to drink plenty of water throughout the day and include hydrating foods such as fruits, vegetables, and herbal teas in your diet.

- **Incorporate Collagen Supplements**: In addition to dietary sources of collagen, you may also consider incorporating collagen supplements into your routine to further support collagen production and promote skin health. Collagen supplements are available in various forms, including powders, capsules, and liquid formulas, and can be easily added to smoothies, beverages, or recipes.

By following these basic principles of the collagen diet and making mindful food choices, you can nourish your body from the inside out, support your body's collagen production, and embrace aging with grace and vitality.

In the next chapters of this cookbook, we'll explore delicious and nutritious recipes specifically designed to support your collagen journey and help you look and feel your best at any age. So get ready to ignite your inner glow and let your radiance shine

BREAKFAST RECIPES

Blueberry Collagen Smoothie

Prep Time: 5 mins

Total Time: 5 mins

Servings: 2 glasses

Ingredients:

- 1 cup frozen organic blueberries
- 1/2 cup ice made with filtered or spring water
- 1 cup coconut water or coconut milk
- 1 1/2 cups leafy greens (kale, spinach, etc.)
- 1/2 avocado or 1/4 cup nuts/seeds
- 1 tsp sweetener (optional)
- Optional additions: collagen powder, protein powder, probiotic powder

Directions:

1. Place all ingredients in a blender.
2. Blend until smooth, adding more water if needed to reach desired consistency.
3. Pour into glasses and serve immediately.

Nutritional Information (per serving):

- Calories: 190
- Protein: 6g
- Fat: 10g
- Carbohydrates: 23g
- Fiber: 7g

- Sugar: 12g

Chia Seed Pudding

Prep Time: 5 mins (plus overnight soaking)

Total Time: 5 mins (plus overnight soaking)

Servings: 2

Ingredients:

- 1/4 cup chia seeds

- 1 cup unsweetened almond milk

- 1/2 tsp vanilla extract

- 1 tbsp honey or maple syrup (optional)

- 1/2 cup fresh berries for topping

Directions:

1. In a bowl, mix chia seeds, almond milk, vanilla extract, and sweetener (if using).

2. Cover and refrigerate overnight or for at least 4 hours until thickened.

3. Stir well before serving, and top with fresh berries.

Nutritional Information (per serving):

- Calories: 180

- Protein: 6g

- Fat: 9g

- Carbohydrates: 20g

- Fiber: 12g

- Sugar: 6g

Collagen-Boosting Oatmeal

Prep Time: 2 mins

Total Time: 5 mins

Servings: 1

Ingredients:

- 1/2 cup rolled oats
- 1 cup water or milk of choice
- 1 tbsp collagen powder
- 1 tbsp almond butter
- 1/2 banana, sliced
- 1 tbsp chopped nuts or seeds
- Optional: drizzle of honey or maple syrup

Directions:

1. In a saucepan, bring water or milk to a boil.
2. Stir in rolled oats and reduce heat to low. Cook for 3-5 minutes, stirring occasionally, until thickened.
3. Remove from heat and stir in collagen powder and almond butter.
4. Transfer to a bowl and top with sliced banana, nuts/seeds, and a drizzle of honey or maple syrup if desired.

Nutritional Information (per serving):

- Calories: 350
- Protein: 15g
- Fat: 12g
- Carbohydrates: 45g
- Fiber: 7g
- Sugar: 8g

Spinach and Feta Egg Muffins

Prep Time: 10 mins

Total Time: 25 mins

Servings: 6 muffins

Ingredients:

- 6 eggs
- 1 cup chopped spinach
- 1/4 cup crumbled feta cheese
- Salt and pepper to taste
- Optional: diced bell peppers, onions, tomatoes

Directions:

1. Preheat oven to 350°F (175°C). Grease a muffin tin or line with paper liners.
2. In a bowl, whisk together eggs, spinach, feta cheese, salt, and pepper.
3. Pour egg mixture evenly into muffin cups, filling each about 3/4 full.
4. Bake for 15-20 minutes, or until eggs are set and lightly golden.
5. Remove from oven and let cool slightly before serving.

Nutritional Information (per muffin):

- Calories: 90
- Protein: 7g
- Fat: 6g
- Carbohydrates: 1g
- Fiber: 0g
- Sugar: 0g

Greek Yogurt Parfait

Prep Time: 5 mins

Total Time: 5 mins

Servings: 1

Ingredients:

- 1/2 cup Greek yogurt
- 1/4 cup granola (choose low-sugar options)
- 1/2 cup mixed berries
- 1 tbsp honey or maple syrup (optional)

Directions:

1. In a glass or bowl, layer Greek yogurt, granola, and mixed berries.
2. Drizzle with honey or maple syrup if desired.
3. Serve immediately or refrigerate until ready to eat.

Nutritional Information (per serving):

- Calories: 250
- Protein: 15g
- Fat: 6g
- Carbohydrates: 35g
- Fiber: 5g
- Sugar: 20g

Strawberry Banana Collagen Smoothie

Prep Time: 5 mins

Total Time: 5 mins

Servings: 2 glasses

Ingredients:

- 1 cup frozen organic strawberries
- 1 ripe banana
- 1/2 cup ice made with filtered or spring water
- 1 cup unsweetened almond milk
- 1 scoop collagen powder
- 1 tbsp almond butter
- Optional: 1 tsp honey or maple syrup for sweetness

Directions:

1. In a blender, combine frozen strawberries, banana, ice, almond milk, collagen powder, and almond butter.
2. Blend until smooth and creamy.
3. Taste and add sweetener if desired.
4. Pour into glasses and serve immediately.

Nutritional Information (per serving):

- Calories: 220
- Protein: 10g
- Fat: 7g
- Carbohydrates: 35g
- Fiber: 8g
- Sugar: 17g

Vanilla Protein Pancakes

Prep Time: 10 mins

Total Time: 20 mins

Servings: 2 servings (about 6 pancakes)

Ingredients:

- 1 cup oat flour

- 1 scoop vanilla protein powder
- 1 tsp baking powder
- 1/2 tsp cinnamon
- 1 ripe banana, mashed
- 1/2 cup unsweetened almond milk
- 1 egg
- 1 tsp vanilla extract
- Optional toppings: fresh berries, almond butter, honey

Directions:

1. In a bowl, whisk together oat flour, protein powder, baking powder, and cinnamon.
2. In a separate bowl, mash the banana and whisk in almond milk, egg, and vanilla extract.
3. Pour wet ingredients into dry ingredients and mix until well combined.
4. Heat a non-stick skillet over medium heat and lightly grease with oil or cooking spray.
5. Pour 1/4 cup of batter onto the skillet for each pancake.
6. Cook until bubbles form on the surface, then flip and cook until golden brown on the other side.
7. Serve warm with your favorite toppings.

Nutritional Information (per serving, 3 pancakes):

- Calories: 320
- Protein: 18g
- Fat: 7g
- Carbohydrates: 45g

- Fiber: 6g

- Sugar: 9g

Collagen-Boosting Acai Bowl

Prep Time: 5 mins

Total Time: 5 mins

Servings: 1

Ingredients:

- 1 pack frozen acai puree

- 1/2 cup frozen mixed berries

- 1/2 banana

- 1/2 cup unsweetened almond milk

- 1 scoop collagen powder

- Toppings: granola, sliced banana, shredded coconut, chia seeds

Directions:

1. In a blender, combine frozen acai puree, mixed berries, banana, almond milk, and collagen powder.

2. Blend until smooth and creamy.

3. Pour into a bowl and add desired toppings.

Nutritional Information (per serving):

- Calories: 320

- Protein: 15g

- Fat: 10g

- Carbohydrates: 50g

- Fiber: 10g

- Sugar: 20g

Avocado Toast with Smoked Salmon

Prep Time: 5 mins

Total Time: 5 mins

Servings: 1

Ingredients:

- 2 slices whole grain bread, toasted
- 1/2 avocado, mashed
- 2 oz. smoked salmon
- 1 tbsp chopped chives or green onions
- Salt and pepper to taste

Directions:

1. Spread mashed avocado evenly on toasted bread slices.
2. Top with smoked salmon and sprinkle with chopped chives or green onions.
3. Season with salt and pepper to taste.

Nutritional Information (per serving):

- Calories: 320
- Protein: 20g
- Fat: 15g
- Carbohydrates: 30g
- Fiber: 10g
- Sugar: 2g

Coconut Chia Seed Pudding

Prep Time: 5 mins (plus overnight soaking)

Total Time: 5 mins (plus overnight soaking)

Servings: 2

Ingredients:

- 1/4 cup chia seeds
- 1 cup coconut milk
- 1/2 tsp vanilla extract
- 1 tbsp honey or maple syrup (optional)
- Fresh fruit for topping

Directions:

1. In a bowl, mix chia seeds, coconut milk, vanilla extract, and sweetener (if using).
2. Cover and refrigerate overnight or for at least 4 hours until thickened.
3. Stir well before serving, and top with fresh fruit.

Nutritional Information (per serving):

- Calories: 250
- Protein: 5g
- Fat: 20g
- Carbohydrates: 15g
- Fiber: 10g
- Sugar: 5g

Protein-Packed Green Smoothie Bowl

Prep Time: 5 mins

Total Time: 5 mins

Servings: 1 bowl

Ingredients:

- 1 frozen banana
- 1 cup frozen organic spinach

- 1 scoop collagen powder
- 1 tbsp almond butter
- 1/2 cup unsweetened almond milk
- Toppings: sliced banana, berries, granola, chia seeds

Directions:

1. In a blender, combine frozen banana, frozen spinach, collagen powder, almond butter, and almond milk.
2. Blend until smooth and creamy.
3. Pour into a bowl and add desired toppings.

Nutritional Information (per serving):

- Calories: 300
- Protein: 15g
- Fat: 10g
- Carbohydrates: 40g
- Fiber: 10g
- Sugar: 20g

Coconut Collagen Chia Pudding

Prep Time: 5 mins (plus overnight soaking)

Total Time: 5 mins (plus overnight soaking)

Servings: 2

Ingredients:

- 1/4 cup chia seeds
- 1 cup coconut milk
- 1 scoop collagen powder
- 1/2 tsp vanilla extract
- 1 tbsp honey or maple syrup (optional)

- Toppings: sliced mango, shredded coconut, chopped nuts

Directions:

1. In a bowl, mix chia seeds, coconut milk, collagen powder, vanilla extract, and sweetener (if using).
2. Cover and refrigerate overnight or for at least 4 hours until thickened.
3. Stir well before serving, and top with desired toppings.

Nutritional Information (per serving):

- Calories: 250
- Protein: 10g
- Fat: 15g
- Carbohydrates: 25g
- Fiber: 10g
- Sugar: 10g

Protein-Packed Oatmeal

Prep Time: 2 mins

Total Time: 5 mins

Servings: 1

Ingredients:

- 1/2 cup rolled oats
- 1 cup water or milk of choice
- 1 scoop collagen powder
- 1 tbsp almond butter
- 1/2 cup mixed berries
- Optional: drizzle of honey or maple syrup

Directions:

1. In a saucepan, bring water or milk to a boil.
2. Stir in rolled oats and reduce heat to low. Cook for 3-5 minutes, stirring occasionally, until thickened.
3. Remove from heat and stir in collagen powder and almond butter.
4. Transfer to a bowl and top with mixed berries and a drizzle of honey or maple syrup if desired.

Nutritional Information (per serving):

- Calories: 350
- Protein: 15g
- Fat: 10g
- Carbohydrates: 45g
- Fiber: 8g
- Sugar: 10g

Greek Yogurt Parfait with Collagen

Prep Time: 5 mins

Total Time: 5 mins

Servings: 1

Ingredients:

- 1/2 cup Greek yogurt
- 1 scoop collagen powder
- 1/4 cup granola (choose low-sugar options)
- 1/2 cup mixed berries
- Optional: drizzle of honey or maple syrup

Directions:

1. In a bowl, mix Greek yogurt and collagen powder until well combined.

2. Layer Greek yogurt mixture with granola and mixed berries.

3. Drizzle with honey or maple syrup if desired.

4. Serve immediately.

Nutritional Information (per serving):

- Calories: 300

- Protein: 25g

- Fat: 5g

- Carbohydrates: 40g

- Fiber: 8g

- Sugar: 20g

Avocado and Egg Breakfast Bowl

Prep Time: 5 mins

Total Time: 10 mins

Servings: 1

Ingredients:

- 1 ripe avocado

- 2 eggs

- 1/4 cup cherry tomatoes, halved

- 1/4 cup diced cucumber

- 1 tbsp chopped fresh herbs (parsley, cilantro)

- Salt and pepper to taste

Directions:

1. Cut the avocado in half and remove the pit. Scoop out some flesh to create a larger well for the eggs.

2. Crack one egg into each avocado half.

3. Place avocado halves on a baking sheet and bake at 375°F (190°C) for 10-15 minutes, or until eggs are cooked to your desired doneness.

4. Remove from oven and top with cherry tomatoes, cucumber, fresh herbs, salt, and pepper.

Nutritional Information (per serving):

- Calories: 320
- Protein: 15g
- Fat: 25g
- Carbohydrates: 15g
- Fiber: 10g
- Sugar: 2g

Vitality Berry Smoothie Bowl

Prep Time: 5 mins

Total Time: 5 mins

Servings: 1 bowl

Ingredients:

- 1 cup frozen mixed berries (blueberries, strawberries, raspberries)
- 1/2 frozen banana
- 1/2 cup unsweetened almond milk
- 1 scoop collagen powder
- 1 tbsp almond butter
- Toppings: sliced strawberries, blueberries, granola, shredded coconut

Directions:

1. In a blender, combine frozen mixed berries, banana, almond milk, collagen powder, and almond butter.
2. Blend until smooth and creamy.
3. Pour into a bowl and add desired toppings.

Nutritional Information (per serving):

- Calories: 300
- Protein: 15g
- Fat: 10g
- Carbohydrates: 40g
- Fiber: 8g
- Sugar: 20g

Collagen-Boosting Green Smoothie

Prep Time: 5 mins

Total Time: 5 mins

Servings: 2 glasses

Ingredients:

- 1 cup frozen organic spinach
- 1/2 cup frozen pineapple chunks
- 1/2 frozen banana
- 1 cup coconut water
- 1 scoop collagen powder
- 1 tbsp chia seeds
- Optional: 1 tsp honey or maple syrup for sweetness

Directions:

1. In a blender, combine frozen spinach, pineapple chunks, banana, coconut water, collagen powder, and chia seeds.
2. Blend until smooth and creamy.
3. Taste and add sweetener if desired.
4. Pour into glasses and serve immediately.

Nutritional Information (per serving):

- Calories: 200
- Protein: 10g
- Fat: 5g
- Carbohydrates: 30g
- Fiber: 8g
- Sugar: 15g

Protein-Packed Greek Yogurt Bowl

Prep Time: 5 mins

Total Time: 5 mins

Servings: 1

Ingredients:

- 1/2 cup Greek yogurt
- 1 scoop collagen powder
- 1/4 cup granola (choose low-sugar options)
- 1/2 cup mixed berries
- Optional: drizzle of honey or maple syrup

Directions:

1. In a bowl, mix Greek yogurt and collagen powder until well combined.
2. Top with granola and mixed berries.

3. Drizzle with honey or maple syrup if desired.

4. Serve immediately.

Nutritional Information (per serving):

- Calories: 300

- Protein: 25g

- Fat: 5g

- Carbohydrates: 40g

- Fiber: 8g

- Sugar: 20g

Collagen-Boosting Breakfast Parfait

Prep Time: 5 mins

Total Time: 5 mins

Servings: 1

Ingredients:

- 1/2 cup rolled oats

- 1 cup unsweetened almond milk

- 1 scoop collagen powder

- 1/2 cup mixed berries

- 1 tbsp almond butter

- Optional: drizzle of honey or maple syrup

Directions:

1. In a jar or bowl, layer rolled oats, almond milk, collagen powder, mixed berries, and almond butter.

2. Repeat layers until ingredients are used up.

3. Drizzle with honey or maple syrup if desired.

4. Refrigerate overnight or for at least 4 hours.

5. Enjoy chilled in the morning.

Nutritional Information (per serving):

- Calories: 350
- Protein: 15g
- Fat: 10g
- Carbohydrates: 45g
- Fiber: 8g
- Sugar: 15g

Collagen-Boosting Breakfast Wrap

Prep Time: 10 mins

Total Time: 10 mins

Servings: 1

Ingredients:

- 1 whole grain tortilla
- 2 eggs, scrambled
- 1/4 avocado, sliced
- Handful of spinach leaves
- 1 slice nitrate-free turkey or chicken breast
- 1 tbsp salsa or hot sauce (optional)
- Salt and pepper to taste

Directions:

1. Heat a non-stick skillet over medium heat.
2. Warm the tortilla for 1-2 minutes on each side until lightly toasted.
3. Spread scrambled eggs onto the center of the tortilla.

4. Layer with avocado slices, spinach leaves, and turkey or chicken breast.

5. Season with salt, pepper, and salsa or hot sauce if desired.

6. Fold the sides of the tortilla over the filling to form a wrap.

7. Serve immediately.

Nutritional Information (per serving):

- Calories: 350
- Protein: 20g
- Fat: 15g
- Carbohydrates: 30g
- Fiber: 8g
- Sugar: 2g

SNACKS RECIPES

Collagen-Boosting Energy Balls

Prep Time: 15 mins

Total Time: 15 mins

Servings: 12 balls

Ingredients:

- 1 cup rolled oats
- 1/2 cup almond butter
- 1/4 cup honey or maple syrup
- 1/4 cup collagen powder
- 1/4 cup unsweetened shredded coconut
- 1/4 cup mini chocolate chips or chopped nuts (optional)
- 1 tsp vanilla extract
- Pinch of salt

Directions:

1. In a large bowl, mix together rolled oats, almond butter, honey or maple syrup, collagen powder, shredded coconut, chocolate chips or nuts (if using), vanilla extract, and salt until well combined.
2. Roll the mixture into small balls, about 1 inch in diameter.
3. Place the energy balls on a baking sheet lined with parchment paper.
4. Refrigerate for at least 30 minutes to firm up.
5. Store in an airtight container in the refrigerator for up to two weeks.

Nutritional Information (per serving, 1 ball):

- Calories: 150
- Protein: 5g
- Fat: 8g
- Carbohydrates: 15g
- Fiber: 2g
- Sugar: 8g

Greek Yogurt and Berry Parfait

Prep Time: 5 mins

Total Time: 5 mins

Servings: 1

Ingredients:

- 1/2 cup Greek yogurt
- 1 scoop collagen powder
- 1/4 cup granola (choose low-sugar options)
- 1/2 cup mixed berries
- Optional: drizzle of honey or maple syrup

Directions:

1. In a glass or bowl, layer Greek yogurt and collagen powder until well combined.
2. Top with granola and mixed berries.
3. Drizzle with honey or maple syrup if desired.
4. Serve immediately.

Nutritional Information (per serving):

- Calories: 250
- Protein: 25g

- Fat: 5g

- Carbohydrates: 40g

- Fiber: 8g

- Sugar: 20g

Collagen-Boosting Green Smoothie

Prep Time: 5 mins

Total Time: 5 mins

Servings: 2 glasses

Ingredients:

- 1 cup frozen organic spinach

- 1/2 cup frozen pineapple chunks

- 1/2 frozen banana

- 1 cup coconut water

- 1 scoop collagen powder

- 1 tbsp chia seeds

- Optional: 1 tsp honey or maple syrup for sweetness

Directions:

1. In a blender, combine frozen spinach, pineapple chunks, banana, coconut water, collagen powder, and chia seeds.

2. Blend until smooth and creamy.

3. Taste and add sweetener if desired.

4. Pour into glasses and serve immediately.

Nutritional Information (per serving):

- Calories: 200

- Protein: 10g

- Fat: 5g

- Carbohydrates: 30g

- Fiber: 8g

- Sugar: 15g

Collagen-Boosting Fruit Salad

Prep Time: 10 mins

Total Time: 10 mins

Servings: 4

Ingredients:

- 2 cups mixed berries (strawberries, blueberries, raspberries)

- 1 mango, peeled and diced

- 1 kiwi, peeled and sliced

- 1/2 cup grapes, halved

- 1 scoop collagen powder

- Juice of 1 lime

- Fresh mint leaves for garnish

Directions:

1. In a large bowl, combine mixed berries, mango, kiwi, and grapes.

2. Sprinkle collagen powder over the fruit and drizzle with lime juice.

3. Gently toss until well combined.

4. Garnish with fresh mint leaves before serving.

Nutritional Information (per serving):

- Calories: 120

- Protein: 3g

- Fat: 0g

- Carbohydrates: 30g

- Fiber: 6g

- Sugar: 20g

Collagen-Boosting Veggie Sticks with Hummus

Prep Time: 10 mins

Total Time: 10 mins

Servings: 4

Ingredients:

- 2 carrots, peeled and cut into sticks

- 2 celery stalks, cut into sticks

- 1 cucumber, cut into sticks

- 1 bell pepper, sliced

- 1 cup cherry tomatoes

- 1 scoop collagen powder

- 1 cup hummus

Directions:

1. Arrange carrot sticks, celery sticks, cucumber sticks, bell pepper slices, and cherry tomatoes on a serving platter.

2. Sprinkle collagen powder over the veggies.

3. Serve with hummus for dipping.

Nutritional Information (per serving):

- Calories: 150

- Protein: 5g

- Fat: 5g

- Carbohydrates: 20g

- Fiber: 6g

- Sugar: 8g

Protein-Packed Collagen Energy Bites

Prep Time: 15 mins

Total Time: 15 mins

Servings: 12 bites

Ingredients:

- 1 cup rolled oats
- 1/2 cup almond butter
- 1/4 cup honey or maple syrup
- 1/4 cup collagen powder
- 1/4 cup unsweetened shredded coconut
- 1/4 cup mini chocolate chips or chopped nuts (optional)
- 1 tsp vanilla extract
- Pinch of salt

Directions:

1. In a large bowl, mix together rolled oats, almond butter, honey or maple syrup, collagen powder, shredded coconut, chocolate chips or nuts (if using), vanilla extract, and salt until well combined.
2. Roll the mixture into small balls, about 1 inch in diameter.
3. Place the energy bites on a baking sheet lined with parchment paper.
4. Refrigerate for at least 30 minutes to firm up.
5. Store in an airtight container in the refrigerator for up to two weeks.

Nutritional Information (per serving, 1 bite):

- Calories: 150

- Protein: 5g

- Fat: 8g

- Carbohydrates: 15g

- Fiber: 2g

- Sugar: 8g

Collagen-Boosting Yogurt Parfait

Prep Time: 5 mins

Total Time: 5 mins

Servings: 1

Ingredients:

- 1/2 cup Greek yogurt

- 1 scoop collagen powder

- 1/4 cup granola (choose low-sugar options)

- 1/2 cup mixed berries

- Optional: drizzle of honey or maple syrup

Directions:

1. In a glass or bowl, layer Greek yogurt and collagen powder until well combined.

2. Top with granola and mixed berries.

3. Drizzle with honey or maple syrup if desired.

4. Serve immediately.

Nutritional Information (per serving):

- Calories: 250

- Protein: 25g

- Fat: 5g

- Carbohydrates: 40g

- Fiber: 8g

- Sugar: 20g

Collagen-Boosting Green Smoothie Bowl

Prep Time: 5 mins

Total Time: 5 mins

Servings: 1 bowl

Ingredients:

- 1 cup frozen organic spinach

- 1/2 frozen banana

- 1/2 cup unsweetened almond milk

- 1 scoop collagen powder

- 1 tbsp almond butter

- Toppings: sliced banana, berries, granola, chia seeds

Directions:

1. In a blender, combine frozen spinach, banana, almond milk, collagen powder, and almond butter.

2. Blend until smooth and creamy.

3. Pour into a bowl and add desired toppings.

Nutritional Information (per serving):

- Calories: 300

- Protein: 15g

- Fat: 10g

- Carbohydrates: 40g

- Fiber: 8g

- Sugar: 20g

Collagen-Boosting Fruit Salad

Prep Time: 10 mins

Total Time: 10 mins

Servings: 4

Ingredients:

- 2 cups mixed berries (strawberries, blueberries, raspberries)
- 1 mango, peeled and diced
- 1 kiwi, peeled and sliced
- 1/2 cup grapes, halved
- 1 scoop collagen powder
- Juice of 1 lime
- Fresh mint leaves for garnish

Directions:

1. In a large bowl, combine mixed berries, mango, kiwi, and grapes.
2. Sprinkle collagen powder over the fruit and drizzle with lime juice.
3. Gently toss until well combined.
4. Garnish with fresh mint leaves before serving.

Nutritional Information (per serving):

- Calories: 120
- Protein: 3g
- Fat: 0g
- Carbohydrates: 30g
- Fiber: 6g
- Sugar: 20g

Collagen-Boosting Veggie Sticks with Hummus

Prep Time: 10 mins

Total Time: 10 mins

Servings: 4

Ingredients:

- 2 carrots, peeled and cut into sticks
- 2 celery stalks, cut into sticks
- 1 cucumber, cut into sticks
- 1 bell pepper, sliced
- 1 cup cherry tomatoes
- 1 scoop collagen powder
- 1 cup hummus

Directions:

1. Arrange carrot sticks, celery sticks, cucumber sticks, bell pepper slices, and cherry tomatoes on a serving platter.
2. Sprinkle collagen powder over the veggies.
3. Serve with hummus for dipping.

Nutritional Information (per serving):

- Calories: 150
- Protein: 5g
- Fat: 5g
- Carbohydrates: 20g
- Fiber: 6g
- Sugar: 8g

Collagen-Boosting Protein Balls

Prep Time: 15 mins

Total Time: 15 mins

Servings: 12 balls

Ingredients:

- 1 cup rolled oats
- 1/2 cup almond butter
- 1/4 cup honey or maple syrup
- 1/4 cup collagen powder
- 1/4 cup unsweetened shredded coconut
- 1/4 cup mini chocolate chips or chopped nuts (optional)
- 1 tsp vanilla extract
- Pinch of salt

Directions:

1. In a large bowl, mix together rolled oats, almond butter, honey or maple syrup, collagen powder, shredded coconut, chocolate chips or nuts (if using), vanilla extract, and salt until well combined.
2. Roll the mixture into small balls, about 1 inch in diameter.
3. Place the energy bites on a baking sheet lined with parchment paper.
4. Refrigerate for at least 30 minutes to firm up.
5. Store in an airtight container in the refrigerator for up to two weeks.

Nutritional Information (per serving, 1 ball):

- Calories: 150
- Protein: 5g

- Fat: 8g

- Carbohydrates: 15g

- Fiber: 2g

- Sugar: 8g

Collagen-Boosting Greek Yogurt Bowl

Prep Time: 5 mins

Total Time: 5 mins

Servings: 1

Ingredients:

- 1/2 cup Greek yogurt

- 1 scoop collagen powder

- 1/4 cup granola (choose low-sugar options)

- 1/2 cup mixed berries

- Optional: drizzle of honey or maple syrup

Directions:

1. In a glass or bowl, layer Greek yogurt and collagen powder until well combined.

2. Top with granola and mixed berries.

3. Drizzle with honey or maple syrup if desired.

4. Serve immediately.

Nutritional Information (per serving):

- Calories: 250

- Protein: 25g

- Fat: 5g

- Carbohydrates: 40g

- Fiber: 8g

- Sugar: 20g

Collagen-Boosting Green Smoothie Bowl

Prep Time: 5 mins

Total Time: 5 mins

Servings: 1 bowl

Ingredients:

- 1 cup frozen organic spinach
- 1/2 frozen banana
- 1/2 cup unsweetened almond milk
- 1 scoop collagen powder
- 1 tbsp almond butter
- Toppings: sliced banana, berries, granola, chia seeds

Directions:

1. In a blender, combine frozen spinach, banana, almond milk, collagen powder, and almond butter.
2. Blend until smooth and creamy.
3. Pour into a bowl and add desired toppings.

Nutritional Information (per serving):

- Calories: 300
- Protein: 15g
- Fat: 10g
- Carbohydrates: 40g
- Fiber: 8g
- Sugar: 20g

Collagen-Boosting Fruit Salad

Prep Time: 10 mins

Total Time: 10 mins

Servings: 4

Ingredients:

- 2 cups mixed berries (strawberries, blueberries, raspberries)
- 1 mango, peeled and diced
- 1 kiwi, peeled and sliced
- 1/2 cup grapes, halved
- 1 scoop collagen powder
- Juice of 1 lime
- Fresh mint leaves for garnish

Directions:

1. In a large bowl, combine mixed berries, mango, kiwi, and grapes.
2. Sprinkle collagen powder over the fruit and drizzle with lime juice.
3. Gently toss until well combined.
4. Garnish with fresh mint leaves before serving.

Nutritional Information (per serving):

- Calories: 120
- Protein: 3g
- Fat: 0g
- Carbohydrates: 30g
- Fiber: 6g
- Sugar: 20g

Collagen-Boosting Veggie Sticks with Hummus

Prep Time: 10 mins

Total Time: 10 mins

Servings: 4

Ingredients:

- 2 carrots, peeled and cut into sticks
- 2 celery stalks, cut into sticks
- 1 cucumber, cut into sticks
- 1 bell pepper, sliced
- 1 cup cherry tomatoes
- 1 scoop collagen powder
- 1 cup hummus

Directions:

1. Arrange carrot sticks, celery sticks, cucumber sticks, bell pepper slices, and cherry tomatoes on a serving platter.
2. Sprinkle collagen powder over the veggies.
3. Serve with hummus for dipping.

Nutritional Information (per serving):

- Calories: 150
- Protein: 5g
- Fat: 5g
- Carbohydrates: 20g
- Fiber: 6g
- Sugar: 8g

Protein-Packed Collagen Energy Balls

- **Prep Time:** 15 mins
- **Total Time:** 15 mins

- **Servings:** 12 balls

Ingredients:

- 1 cup rolled oats
- 1/2 cup almond butter
- 1/4 cup honey or maple syrup
- 1/4 cup collagen powder
- 1/4 cup unsweetened shredded coconut
- 1/4 cup mini chocolate chips or chopped nuts (optional)
- 1 tsp vanilla extract
- Pinch of salt

Directions:

1. In a large bowl, mix together rolled oats, almond butter, honey or maple syrup, collagen powder, shredded coconut, chocolate chips or nuts (if using), vanilla extract, and salt until well combined.
2. Roll the mixture into small balls, about 1 inch in diameter.
3. Place the energy bites on a baking sheet lined with parchment paper.
4. Refrigerate for at least 30 minutes to firm up.
5. Store in an airtight container in the refrigerator for up to two weeks.

Nutritional Information (per serving, 1 ball):

- Calories: 150
- Protein: 5g
- Fat: 8g
- Carbohydrates: 15g

- Fiber: 2g
- Sugar: 8g

Collagen-Infused Greek Yogurt Parfait

Prep Time: 5 mins

Total Time: 5 mins

Servings: 1

Ingredients:

- 1/2 cup Greek yogurt
- 1 scoop collagen powder
- 1/4 cup granola (choose low-sugar options)
- 1/2 cup mixed berries
- Optional: drizzle of honey or maple syrup

Directions:

1. In a glass or bowl, layer Greek yogurt and collagen powder until well combined.
2. Top with granola and mixed berries.
3. Drizzle with honey or maple syrup if desired.
4. Serve immediately.

Nutritional Information (per serving):

- Calories: 250
- Protein: 25g
- Fat: 5g
- Carbohydrates: 40g
- Fiber: 8g
- Sugar: 20g

Green Collagen Smoothie Bowl

Prep Time: 5 mins

Total Time: 5 mins

Servings: 1 bowl

Ingredients:

- 1 cup frozen organic spinach
- 1/2 frozen banana
- 1/2 cup unsweetened almond milk
- 1 scoop collagen powder
- 1 tbsp almond butter
- Toppings: sliced banana, berries, granola, chia seeds

Directions:

1. In a blender, combine frozen spinach, banana, almond milk, collagen powder, and almond butter.
2. Blend until smooth and creamy.
3. Pour into a bowl and add desired toppings.

Nutritional Information (per serving):

- Calories: 300
- Protein: 15g
- Fat: 10g
- Carbohydrates: 40g
- Fiber: 8g
- Sugar: 20g

Mixed Berry Collagen Fruit Salad

Prep Time: 10 mins

Total Time: 10 mins

Servings: 4

Ingredients:

- 2 cups mixed berries (strawberries, blueberries, raspberries)
- 1 mango, peeled and diced
- 1 kiwi, peeled and sliced
- 1/2 cup grapes, halved
- 1 scoop collagen powder
- Juice of 1 lime
- Fresh mint leaves for garnish

Directions:

1. In a large bowl, combine mixed berries, mango, kiwi, and grapes.
2. Sprinkle collagen powder over the fruit and drizzle with lime juice.
3. Gently toss until well combined.
4. Garnish with fresh mint leaves before serving.

Nutritional Information (per serving):

- Calories: 120
- Protein: 3g
- Fat: 0g
- Carbohydrates: 30g
- Fiber: 6g
- Sugar: 20g

Veggie Sticks with Collagen-Enhanced Hummus

Prep Time: 10 mins

Total Time: 10 mins

Servings: 4

Ingredients:

- 2 carrots, peeled and cut into sticks
- 2 celery stalks, cut into sticks
- 1 cucumber, cut into sticks
- 1 bell pepper, sliced
- 1 cup cherry tomatoes
- 1 scoop collagen powder
- 1 cup hummus

Directions:

1. Arrange carrot sticks, celery sticks, cucumber sticks, bell pepper slices, and cherry tomatoes on a serving platter.
2. Sprinkle collagen powder over the veggies.
3. Serve with hummus for dipping.

Nutritional Information (per serving):

- Calories: 150
- Protein: 5g
- Fat: 5g
- Carbohydrates: 20g
- Fiber: 6g
- Sugar: 8g

SOUP RECIPES

Nourishing Chicken Bone Broth Soup

Prep Time: 10 mins

Cook Time: 8-12 hours (slow cooker) or 2-3 hours (stovetop)

Total Time: 8-12 hours (slow cooker) or 2-3 hours (stovetop)

Servings: 4

Ingredients:

- 2 lbs chicken bones (preferably with some meat attached)
- 1 onion, quartered
- 2 carrots, chopped
- 2 celery stalks, chopped
- 4 cloves garlic, smashed
- 1 tbsp apple cider vinegar
- Handful of fresh parsley
- Salt and pepper to taste
- Water

Directions:

1. Place chicken bones, onion, carrots, celery, garlic, apple cider vinegar, parsley, salt, and pepper in a slow cooker or large pot.
2. Cover with water, leaving about an inch of space at the top.
3. If using a slow cooker, cook on low for 8-12 hours. If using a stovetop, bring to a boil, then reduce heat and simmer for 2-3 hours.
4. Once cooked, strain the broth to remove solids.
5. Serve hot, optionally garnished with fresh herbs.

Nutritional Information (per serving):

- Calories: 50
- Protein: 6g
- Fat: 2g
- Carbohydrates: 3g
- Fiber: 1g
- Sugar: 1g

Creamy Mushroom Collagen Soup

Prep Time: 10 mins

Cook Time: 20 mins

Total Time: 30 mins

Servings: 4

Ingredients:

- 1 tbsp olive oil
- 1 onion, diced
- 2 cloves garlic, minced
- 8 oz. mushrooms, sliced
- 4 cups vegetable or chicken broth
- 1 scoop collagen powder
- 1/2 cup heavy cream or coconut cream
- Salt and pepper to taste
- Fresh parsley for garnish

Directions:

1. Heat olive oil in a large pot over medium heat. Add onion and garlic, sauté until softened.
2. Add mushrooms and cook until browned and tender.

3. Pour in broth and bring to a simmer.

4. Stir in collagen powder until dissolved.

5. Reduce heat and stir in cream. Simmer for an additional 5 minutes.

6. Season with salt and pepper to taste.

7. Serve hot, garnished with fresh parsley.

Nutritional Information (per serving):

- Calories: 150

- Protein: 5g

- Fat: 10g

- Carbohydrates: 10g

- Fiber: 2g

- Sugar: 4g

Turmeric Lentil Collagen Soup

Prep Time: 10 mins

Cook Time: 30 mins

Total Time: 40 mins

Servings: 6

Ingredients:

- 1 tbsp olive oil

- 1 onion, diced

- 2 cloves garlic, minced

- 1 tsp ground turmeric

- 1 cup dried red lentils

- 4 cups vegetable broth

- 1 scoop collagen powder

- Salt and pepper to taste
- Fresh cilantro for garnish

Directions:

1. Heat olive oil in a large pot over medium heat. Add onion and garlic, sauté until softened.
2. Stir in ground turmeric and cook for 1 minute.
3. Add lentils and broth. Bring to a boil, then reduce heat and simmer for 20-25 minutes, or until lentils are tender.
4. Stir in collagen powder until dissolved.
5. Season with salt and pepper to taste.
6. Serve hot, garnished with fresh cilantro.

Nutritional Information (per serving):

- Calories: 200
- Protein: 10g
- Fat: 3g
- Carbohydrates: 30g
- Fiber: 8g
- Sugar: 3g

Coconut Curry Collagen Soup

Prep Time: 10 mins

Cook Time: 20 mins

Total Time: 30 mins

Servings: 4

Ingredients:

- 1 tbsp coconut oil
- 1 onion, diced

- 2 cloves garlic, minced
- 1 tbsp curry powder
- 1 can (14 oz) coconut milk
- 4 cups vegetable or chicken broth
- 1 scoop collagen powder
- 2 cups diced vegetables (such as bell peppers, carrots, and zucchini)
- Salt and pepper to taste
- Fresh cilantro for garnish

Directions:

1. Heat coconut oil in a large pot over medium heat. Add onion and garlic, sauté until softened.
2. Stir in curry powder and cook for 1 minute.
3. Pour in coconut milk and broth. Bring to a simmer.
4. Add collagen powder and stir until dissolved.
5. Add diced vegetables and simmer for 10-15 minutes, or until vegetables are tender.
6. Season with salt and pepper to taste.
7. Serve hot, garnished with fresh cilantro.

Nutritional Information (per serving):

- Calories: 250
- Protein: 5g
- Fat: 20g
- Carbohydrates: 15g
- Fiber: 5g
- Sugar: 5g

Hearty Vegetable and Quinoa Collagen Soup

Prep Time: 15 mins

Cook Time: 25 mins

Total Time: 40 mins

Servings: 6

Ingredients:

- 1 tbsp olive oil
- 1 onion, diced
- 2 cloves garlic, minced
- 2 carrots, diced
- 2 celery stalks, diced
- 1 cup quinoa, rinsed
- 6 cups vegetable or chicken broth
- 1 scoop collagen powder
- 2 cups chopped kale or spinach
- Salt and pepper to taste
- Fresh parsley for garnish

Directions:

1. Heat olive oil in a large pot over medium heat. Add onion and garlic, sauté until softened.
2. Add carrots and celery, cook for 5 minutes.
3. Stir in quinoa and broth. Bring to a boil, then reduce heat and simmer for 15-20 minutes, or until quinoa is cooked.
4. Stir in collagen powder until dissolved.
5. Add chopped kale or spinach and cook until wilted.
6. Season with salt and pepper to taste.

7. Serve hot, garnished with fresh parsley.

Nutritional Information (per serving):

- Calories: 200
- Protein: 8g
- Fat: 5g
- Carbohydrates: 30g
- Fiber: 5g
- Sugar: 5g

Lemon Chicken Collagen Soup

Prep Time: 15 mins

Cook Time: 30 mins

Total Time: 45 mins

Servings: 4

Ingredients:

- 1 tbsp olive oil
- 1 onion, diced
- 2 cloves garlic, minced
- 2 carrots, sliced
- 2 celery stalks, sliced
- 6 cups chicken broth
- 1 lb boneless, skinless chicken breasts, cut into bite-sized pieces
- Juice of 1 lemon
- 1 scoop collagen powder
- Salt and pepper to taste
- Fresh parsley for garnish

Directions:

1. Heat olive oil in a large pot over medium heat. Add onion and garlic, sauté until softened.
2. Add carrots and celery, cook for 5 minutes.
3. Pour in chicken broth and bring to a simmer.
4. Add chicken pieces and cook for 10-15 minutes, or until cooked through.
5. Stir in lemon juice and collagen powder until dissolved.
6. Season with salt and pepper to taste.
7. Serve hot, garnished with fresh parsley.

Nutritional Information (per serving):

- Calories: 200
- Protein: 25g
- Fat: 5g
- Carbohydrates: 10g
- Fiber: 2g
- Sugar: 3g

Tomato Basil Collagen Soup

Prep Time: 10 mins

Cook Time: 30 mins

Total Time: 40 mins

Servings: 4

Ingredients:

- 1 tbsp olive oil
- 1 onion, diced
- 2 cloves garlic, minced
- 4 cups vegetable broth

- 1 can (28 oz) diced tomatoes
- 1 scoop collagen powder
- 1/4 cup fresh basil leaves, chopped
- Salt and pepper to taste
- Grated Parmesan cheese for garnish (optional)

Directions:

1. Heat olive oil in a large pot over medium heat. Add onion and garlic, sauté until softened.
2. Add vegetable broth and diced tomatoes (with juices). Bring to a simmer.
3. Stir in collagen powder until dissolved.
4. Simmer for 20-25 minutes, stirring occasionally.
5. Stir in fresh basil and season with salt and pepper to taste.
6. Serve hot, garnished with grated Parmesan cheese if desired.

Nutritional Information (per serving):

- Calories: 150
- Protein: 5g
- Fat: 5g
- Carbohydrates: 20g
- Fiber: 5g
- Sugar: 8g

Spicy Pumpkin Collagen Soup

Prep Time: 10 mins

Cook Time: 25 mins

Total Time: 35 mins

Servings: 4

Ingredients:

- 1 tbsp coconut oil
- 1 onion, diced
- 2 cloves garlic, minced
- 1 can (15 oz) pumpkin puree
- 4 cups vegetable broth
- 1 scoop collagen powder
- 1/2 tsp ground cinnamon
- 1/2 tsp ground cumin
- 1/4 tsp cayenne pepper
- Salt and pepper to taste
- Greek yogurt or coconut cream for garnish (optional)

Directions:

1. Heat coconut oil in a large pot over medium heat. Add onion and garlic, sauté until softened.
2. Stir in pumpkin puree, vegetable broth, collagen powder, cinnamon, cumin, and cayenne pepper.
3. Bring to a simmer and cook for 15-20 minutes, stirring occasionally.
4. Season with salt and pepper to taste.
5. Serve hot, garnished with a dollop of Greek yogurt or coconut cream if desired.

Nutritional Information (per serving):

- Calories: 120
- Protein: 5g
- Fat: 5g

- Carbohydrates: 15g

- Fiber: 5g

- Sugar: 5g

Broccoli Cheddar Collagen Soup

Prep Time: 10 mins

Cook Time: 20 mins

Total Time: 30 mins

Servings: 4

Ingredients:

- 2 tbsp butter

- 1 onion, diced

- 2 cloves garlic, minced

- 4 cups vegetable or chicken broth

- 1 large head of broccoli, chopped

- 1 scoop collagen powder

- 1 cup shredded cheddar cheese

- Salt and pepper to taste

Directions:

1. In a large pot, melt butter over medium heat. Add onion and garlic, sauté until softened.

2. Pour in broth and bring to a simmer.

3. Add chopped broccoli and cook for 10-15 minutes, or until tender.

4. Stir in collagen powder until dissolved.

5. Using an immersion blender or regular blender, blend the soup until smooth.

6. Return the soup to the pot and stir in shredded cheddar cheese until melted and smooth.

7. Season with salt and pepper to taste.

8. Serve hot.

Nutritional Information (per serving):

- Calories: 250

- Protein: 10g

- Fat: 15g

Ginger Carrot Collagen Soup

Prep Time: 10 mins

Cook Time: 25 mins

Total Time: 35 mins

Servings: 4

Ingredients:

- 1 tbsp olive oil

- 1 onion, diced

- 2 cloves garlic, minced

- 1-inch piece of ginger, peeled and minced

- 1 lb carrots, peeled and chopped

- 4 cups vegetable broth

- 1 scoop collagen powder

- Salt and pepper to taste

- Fresh cilantro for garnish

Directions:

1. Heat olive oil in a large pot over medium heat. Add onion, garlic, and ginger, sauté until softened.

2. Add chopped carrots and cook for 5 minutes.

3. Pour in vegetable broth and bring to a simmer. Cook until the carrots are tender, about 15-20 minutes.

4. Stir in collagen powder until dissolved.

5. Using an immersion blender or regular blender, blend the soup until smooth.

6. Season with salt and pepper to taste.

7. Serve hot, garnished with fresh cilantro.

Nutritional Information (per serving):

- Calories: 120
- Protein: 5g
- Fat: 3g
- Carbohydrates: 20g
- Fiber: 5g
- Sugar: 8g

Spinach and Lentil Collagen Soup

Prep Time: 15 mins

Cook Time: 30 mins

Total Time: 45 mins

Servings: 4

Ingredients:

- 1 tbsp olive oil
- 1 onion, diced
- 2 cloves garlic, minced
- 1 cup dried green lentils, rinsed
- 4 cups vegetable broth

- 2 cups fresh spinach leaves
- 1 scoop collagen powder
- Salt and pepper to taste
- Lemon wedges for serving

Directions:

1. Heat olive oil in a large pot over medium heat. Add onion and garlic, sauté until softened.
2. Add dried lentils and vegetable broth. Bring to a boil, then reduce heat and simmer for 20-25 minutes, or until lentils are tender.
3. Stir in fresh spinach leaves and cook until wilted.
4. Stir in collagen powder until dissolved.
5. Season with salt and pepper to taste.
6. Serve hot with lemon wedges for squeezing.

Nutritional Information (per serving):

- Calories: 220
- Protein: 15g
- Fat: 3g
- Carbohydrates: 35g
- Fiber: 15g
- Sugar: 5g

Coconut Lime Collagen Soup

Prep Time: 10 mins

Cook Time: 20 mins

Total Time: 30 mins

Servings: 4

Ingredients:

- 1 tbsp coconut oil
- 1 onion, diced
- 2 cloves garlic, minced
- 1-inch piece of ginger, peeled and minced
- 2 cups sweet potato, peeled and chopped
- 4 cups vegetable broth
- 1 can (14 oz) coconut milk
- Juice and zest of 1 lime
- 1 scoop collagen powder
- Salt and pepper to taste
- Fresh cilantro for garnish

Directions:

1. Heat coconut oil in a large pot over medium heat. Add onion, garlic, and ginger, sauté until softened.
2. Add chopped sweet potato and cook for 5 minutes.
3. Pour in vegetable broth and bring to a simmer. Cook until the sweet potatoes are tender, about 15-20 minutes.
4. Stir in coconut milk, lime juice, lime zest, and collagen powder until dissolved.
5. Season with salt and pepper to taste.
6. Serve hot, garnished with fresh cilantro.

Nutritional Information (per serving):

- Calories: 300
- Protein: 5g
- Fat: 20g

- Carbohydrates: 30g

- Fiber: 5g

- Sugar: 8g

Creamy Cauliflower Collagen Soup

Prep Time: 10 mins

Cook Time: 25 mins

Total Time: 35 mins

Servings: 4

Ingredients:

- 1 tbsp olive oil

- 1 onion, diced

- 2 cloves garlic, minced

- 1 head cauliflower, chopped

- 4 cups vegetable broth

- 1 scoop collagen powder

- Salt and pepper to taste

- Fresh chives for garnish

Directions:

1. Heat olive oil in a large pot over medium heat. Add onion and garlic, sauté until softened.

2. Add chopped cauliflower and vegetable broth. Bring to a boil, then reduce heat and simmer for 15-20 minutes, or until cauliflower is tender.

3. Stir in collagen powder until dissolved.

4. Using an immersion blender or regular blender, blend the soup until smooth.

5. Season with salt and pepper to taste.

6. Serve hot, garnished with fresh chives.

Nutritional Information (per serving):

- Calories: 150

- Protein: 5g

- Fat: 5g

- Carbohydrates: 20g

- Fiber: 5g

- Sugar: 5g

Creamy Mushroom Collagen Soup

- **Prep Time:** 10 mins

- **Cook Time:** 25 mins

- **Total Time:** 35 mins

- **Servings:** 4

Ingredients:

- 2 tbsp olive oil

- 1 onion, finely chopped

- 2 cloves garlic, minced

- 1 lb mushrooms, sliced (button or cremini)

- 4 cups vegetable or chicken broth

- 1 scoop collagen powder

- 1/2 cup heavy cream

- Salt and pepper to taste

- Fresh thyme for garnish

Directions:

1. Heat olive oil in a large pot over medium heat. Add onion and garlic, sauté until softened.
2. Add sliced mushrooms and cook until they release their moisture and begin to brown, about 10 minutes.
3. Pour in the broth and bring to a simmer. Cook for an additional 10 minutes.
4. Stir in collagen powder until dissolved.
5. Remove the pot from heat and use an immersion blender to blend the soup until smooth.
6. Return the pot to low heat, stir in heavy cream, and simmer for 5 minutes.
7. Season with salt and pepper to taste.
8. Serve hot, garnished with fresh thyme leaves.

Nutritional Information (per serving):

- Calories: 200
- Protein: 6g
- Fat: 15g
- Carbohydrates: 10g
- Fiber: 2g
- Sugar: 4g

Roasted Tomato Collagen Soup

- **Prep Time:** 15 mins
- **Cook Time:** 45 mins
- **Total Time:** 1 hour
- **Servings:** 4

Ingredients:

- 1 lb tomatoes, halved
- 2 tbsp olive oil
- Salt and pepper to taste
- 1 onion, diced
- 2 cloves garlic, minced
- 4 cups vegetable broth
- 1 scoop collagen powder
- 2 tbsp fresh basil, chopped
- 2 tbsp heavy cream (optional)

Directions:

1. Preheat the oven to 400°F (200°C). Place halved tomatoes on a baking sheet, drizzle with olive oil, and season with salt and pepper. Roast for 30-35 minutes until softened and slightly charred.
2. In a large pot, heat olive oil over medium heat. Add diced onion and minced garlic, sauté until translucent.
3. Add roasted tomatoes and vegetable broth to the pot. Bring to a boil, then reduce heat and simmer for 15 minutes.
4. Stir in collagen powder until dissolved.
5. Use an immersion blender to blend the soup until smooth.
6. Stir in chopped basil and heavy cream (if using), and simmer for an additional 5 minutes.
7. Season with salt and pepper to taste.
8. Serve hot.

Nutritional Information (per serving):

- Calories: 180

- Protein: 5g

- Fat: 10g

- Carbohydrates: 15g

- Fiber: 4g

- Sugar: 8g

Broccoli and Spinach Collagen Soup

Prep Time: 10 mins

Cook Time: 20 mins

Total Time: 30 mins

Servings: 4

Ingredients:

- 1 tbsp olive oil

- 1 onion, chopped

- 2 cloves garlic, minced

- 1 head broccoli, chopped

- 4 cups vegetable broth

- 2 cups fresh spinach

- 1 scoop collagen powder

- Salt and pepper to taste

- Lemon wedges for serving

Directions:

1. Heat olive oil in a large pot over medium heat. Add chopped onion and minced garlic, sauté until softened.

2. Add chopped broccoli and vegetable broth to the pot. Bring to a boil, then reduce heat and simmer for 10-15 minutes until broccoli is tender.

3. Stir in fresh spinach leaves and cook until wilted.

4. Stir in collagen powder until dissolved.

5. Use an immersion blender to blend the soup until smooth.

6. Season with salt and pepper to taste.

7. Serve hot with lemon wedges for squeezing.

Nutritional Information (per serving):

- Calories: 150

- Protein: 5g

- Fat: 6g

- Carbohydrates: 20g

- Fiber: 5g

- Sugar: 5g

Creamy Cauliflower and Leek Collagen Soup

Prep Time: 10 mins

Cook Time: 25 mins

Total Time: 35 mins

Servings: 4

Ingredients:

- 2 tbsp butter

- 2 leeks, white and light green parts only, chopped

- 1 head cauliflower, chopped

- 4 cups vegetable broth

- 1 scoop collagen powder

- Salt and pepper to taste

- Fresh parsley for garnish

Directions:

1. In a large pot, melt butter over medium heat. Add chopped leeks and sauté until softened.

2. Add chopped cauliflower and vegetable broth to the pot. Bring to a boil, then reduce heat and simmer for 15-20 minutes until cauliflower is tender.

3. Stir in collagen powder until dissolved.

4. Use an immersion blender to blend the soup until smooth.

5. Season with salt and pepper to taste.

6. Serve hot, garnished with fresh parsley.

Nutritional Information (per serving):

- Calories: 160
- Protein: 5g
- Fat: 7g
- Carbohydrates: 20g
- Fiber: 5g
- Sugar: 5g

SALAD RECIPES

Avocado and Quinoa Salad

Prep Time: 15 mins

Total Time: 20 mins

Servings: 2

Ingredients:

- 1 cup cooked quinoa, cooled
- 1 avocado, diced
- 1 cup cherry tomatoes, halved
- 1/4 cup red onion, thinly sliced
- 1/4 cup cucumber, diced
- 2 tbsp fresh cilantro, chopped
- Juice of 1 lime
- 2 tbsp olive oil
- Salt and pepper to taste
- 1 scoop collagen powder (optional)

Directions:

1. In a large bowl, combine cooked quinoa, diced avocado, cherry tomatoes, red onion, cucumber, and fresh cilantro.
2. In a small bowl, whisk together lime juice, olive oil, salt, pepper, and collagen powder (if using).
3. Pour the dressing over the salad and toss gently to combine.
4. Serve immediately.

Nutritional Information (per serving):

- Calories: 350

- Protein: 8g

- Fat: 20g

- Carbohydrates: 35g

- Fiber: 8g

- Sugar: 3g

Kale and Mango Salad

Prep Time: 10 mins

Total Time: 15 mins

Servings: 2

Ingredients:

- 4 cups kale, stems removed and chopped

- 1 mango, diced

- 1/4 cup red bell pepper, thinly sliced

- 1/4 cup red cabbage, shredded

- 1/4 cup carrots, grated

- 2 tbsp pumpkin seeds

- Juice of 1 lemon

- 1 tbsp olive oil

- Salt and pepper to taste

- 1 scoop collagen powder (optional)

Directions:

1. In a large bowl, massage kale with lemon juice and olive oil for a few minutes until slightly softened.

2. Add diced mango, red bell pepper, red cabbage, carrots, and pumpkin seeds to the bowl.

3. If using, sprinkle collagen powder over the salad.

4. Season with salt and pepper to taste.

5. Toss gently to combine.

6. Serve immediately.

Nutritional Information (per serving):

- Calories: 280

- Protein: 6g

- Fat: 12g

- Carbohydrates: 40g

- Fiber: 8g

- Sugar: 18g

Spinach and Strawberry Salad

Prep Time: 10 mins

Total Time: 15 mins

Servings: 2

Ingredients:

- 4 cups fresh spinach leaves

- 1 cup strawberries, sliced

- 1/4 cup feta cheese, crumbled

- 2 tbsp sliced almonds

- 2 tbsp balsamic vinegar

- 1 tbsp olive oil

- Salt and pepper to taste

- 1 scoop collagen powder (optional)

Directions:

1. In a large bowl, combine fresh spinach leaves, sliced strawberries, crumbled feta cheese, and sliced almonds.

2. In a small bowl, whisk together balsamic vinegar, olive oil, salt, pepper, and collagen powder (if using).

3. Drizzle the dressing over the salad and toss gently to combine.

4. Serve immediately.

Nutritional Information (per serving):

- Calories: 220
- Protein: 7g
- Fat: 15g
- Carbohydrates: 18g
- Fiber: 6g
- Sugar: 8g

Greek Chickpea Salad

Prep Time: 10 mins

Total Time: 15 mins

Servings: 2

Ingredients:

- 1 can (15 oz) chickpeas, drained and rinsed
- 1/2 cucumber, diced
- 1/2 cup cherry tomatoes, halved
- 1/4 cup red onion, thinly sliced
- 1/4 cup Kalamata olives, pitted
- 2 tbsp crumbled feta cheese
- 2 tbsp fresh parsley, chopped
- Juice of 1 lemon
- 1 tbsp olive oil
- Salt and pepper to taste

- 1 scoop collagen powder (optional)

Directions:

1. In a large bowl, combine chickpeas, diced cucumber, cherry tomatoes, red onion, Kalamata olives, crumbled feta cheese, and fresh parsley.
2. In a small bowl, whisk together lemon juice, olive oil, salt, pepper, and collagen powder (if using).
3. Pour the dressing over the salad and toss gently to combine.
4. Serve immediately.

Nutritional Information (per serving):

- Calories: 280
- Protein: 9g
- Fat: 12g
- Carbohydrates: 35g
- Fiber: 9g
- Sugar: 7g

Tuna and White Bean Salad

Prep Time: 10 mins

Total Time: 15 mins

Servings: 2

Ingredients:

- 1 can (5 oz) tuna, drained
- 1 can (15 oz) white beans, drained and rinsed
- 1/4 cup red onion, finely chopped
- 1/4 cup celery, finely chopped
- 1/4 cup fresh parsley, chopped

- Juice of 1 lemon
- 2 tbsp olive oil
- Salt and pepper to taste
- 1 scoop collagen powder (optional)

Directions:

1. In a large bowl, combine drained tuna, white beans, chopped red onion, chopped celery, and chopped parsley.
2. In a small bowl, whisk together lemon juice, olive oil, salt, pepper, and collagen powder (if using).
3. Pour the dressing over the salad and toss gently to combine.
4. Serve immediately.

Nutritional Information (per serving):

- Calories: 320
- Protein: 18g
- Fat: 14g
- Carbohydrates: 30g
- Fiber: 9g
- Sugar: 2g

Mango Chicken Salad

Prep Time: 15 mins

Total Time: 20 mins

Servings: 2

Ingredients:

- 2 boneless, skinless chicken breasts
- 4 cups mixed greens (e.g., kale, spinach, arugula)
- 1 mango, diced

- 1/4 cup red bell pepper, diced
- 1/4 cup red onion, thinly sliced
- 1/4 cup cucumber, sliced
- 2 tbsp chopped fresh cilantro
- Juice of 1 lime
- 2 tbsp olive oil
- Salt and pepper to taste
- 1 scoop collagen powder (optional)

Directions:

1. Season chicken breasts with salt and pepper. Grill or pan-sear until fully cooked, about 6-8 minutes per side. Let cool, then slice into strips.
2. In a large bowl, combine mixed greens, diced mango, diced red bell pepper, sliced red onion, sliced cucumber, and chopped fresh cilantro.
3. In a small bowl, whisk together lime juice, olive oil, salt, pepper, and collagen powder (if using).
4. Add the sliced chicken to the salad, then drizzle the dressing over the salad mixture.
5. Toss gently to combine.
6. Serve immediately.

Nutritional Information (per serving):

- Calories: 320
- Protein: 30g
- Fat: 15g
- Carbohydrates: 20g

- Fiber: 5g

- Sugar: 10g

Tuna and Avocado Salad

Prep Time: 10 mins

Total Time: 15 mins

Servings: 2

Ingredients:

- 1 can (5 oz) tuna, drained

- 1 avocado, diced

- 4 cups mixed greens (e.g., spinach, romaine, lettuce)

- 1/4 cup cherry tomatoes, halved

- 1/4 cup cucumber, diced

- 2 tbsp sliced almonds

- Juice of 1 lemon

- 2 tbsp olive oil

- Salt and pepper to taste

- 1 scoop collagen powder (optional)

Directions:

1. In a large bowl, combine drained tuna, diced avocado, mixed greens, halved cherry tomatoes, diced cucumber, and sliced almonds.

2. In a small bowl, whisk together lemon juice, olive oil, salt, pepper, and collagen powder (if using).

3. Pour the dressing over the salad mixture.

4. Toss gently to combine.

5. Serve immediately.

Nutritional Information (per serving):

- Calories: 350
- Protein: 25g
- Fat: 25g
- Carbohydrates: 15g
- Fiber: 7g
- Sugar: 5g

Quinoa and Black Bean Salad

Prep Time: 15 mins

Total Time: 20 mins

Servings: 2

Ingredients:

- 1 cup cooked quinoa, cooled
- 1 can (15 oz) black beans, drained and rinsed
- 4 cups mixed greens (e.g., kale, arugula, chard)
- 1/4 cup red onion, thinly sliced
- 1/4 cup corn kernels (fresh or frozen)
- 1/4 cup diced bell pepper (any color)
- 2 tbsp chopped fresh cilantro
- Juice of 1 lime
- 2 tbsp olive oil
- Salt and pepper to taste
- 1 scoop collagen powder (optional)

Directions:

1. In a large bowl, combine cooked quinoa, black beans, mixed greens, sliced red onion, corn kernels, diced bell pepper, and chopped fresh cilantro.

2. In a small bowl, whisk together lime juice, olive oil, salt, pepper, and collagen powder (if using).

3. Pour the dressing over the salad mixture.

4. Toss gently to combine.

5. Serve immediately.

Nutritional Information (per serving):

- Calories: 320
- Protein: 15g
- Fat: 10g
- Carbohydrates: 45g
- Fiber: 12g
- Sugar: 5g

Asian-Inspired Salmon Salad

Prep Time: 10 mins

Total Time: 20 mins

Servings: 2

Ingredients:

- 2 salmon fillets
- 4 cups mixed greens (e.g., spinach, cabbage, lettuce)
- 1/4 cup shredded carrots
- 1/4 cup sliced cucumber
- 1/4 cup edamame (cooked and shelled)
- 2 tbsp sliced almonds

- 2 tbsp sesame seeds
- 2 tbsp soy sauce
- 1 tbsp rice vinegar
- 1 tbsp sesame oil
- 1 tsp honey
- 1 scoop collagen powder (optional)

Directions:

1. Season salmon fillets with salt and pepper. Grill or bake until fully cooked, about 10-12 minutes. Let cool, then flake into bite-sized pieces.
2. In a large bowl, combine mixed greens, shredded carrots, sliced cucumber, edamame, sliced almonds, and sesame seeds.
3. In a small bowl, whisk together soy sauce, rice vinegar, sesame oil, honey, and collagen powder (if using).
4. Add the flaked salmon to the salad, then drizzle the dressing over the salad mixture.
5. Toss gently to combine.
6. Serve immediately.

Nutritional Information (per serving):

- Calories: 380
- Protein: 30g
- Fat: 20g
- Carbohydrates: 20g
- Fiber: 6

Berry Spinach Salad

Prep Time: 10 mins

Total Time: 10 mins

Servings: 2

Ingredients:

- 4 cups baby spinach
- 1 cup mixed berries (e.g., strawberries, blueberries, raspberries)
- 1/4 cup sliced almonds
- 1/4 cup crumbled feta cheese
- 2 tbsp balsamic vinegar
- 2 tbsp olive oil
- Salt and pepper to taste
- 1 scoop collagen powder (optional)

Directions:

1. In a large bowl, combine baby spinach, mixed berries, sliced almonds, and crumbled feta cheese.
2. In a small bowl, whisk together balsamic vinegar, olive oil, salt, pepper, and collagen powder (if using).
3. Drizzle the dressing over the salad mixture.
4. Toss gently to combine.
5. Serve immediately.

Nutritional Information (per serving):

- Calories: 230
- Protein: 7g
- Fat: 16g
- Carbohydrates: 17g
- Fiber: 6g
- Sugar: 7g

Chicken Caesar Salad

Prep Time: 15 mins

Total Time: 15 mins

Servings: 2

Ingredients:

- 2 boneless, skinless chicken breasts
- 4 cups romaine lettuce, chopped
- 1/4 cup grated Parmesan cheese
- 1/4 cup Caesar dressing
- 1/4 cup croutons
- Juice of 1 lemon
- Salt and pepper to taste
- 1 scoop collagen powder (optional)

Directions:

1. Season chicken breasts with salt and pepper. Grill or pan-sear until fully cooked, about 6-8 minutes per side. Let cool, then slice into strips.
2. In a large bowl, combine chopped romaine lettuce, grated Parmesan cheese, and croutons.
3. Add the sliced chicken to the salad.
4. Drizzle Caesar dressing over the salad mixture.
5. Squeeze lemon juice over the salad.
6. Toss gently to combine.
7. Serve immediately.

Nutritional Information (per serving):

- Calories: 340

- Protein: 35g
- Fat: 18g
- Carbohydrates: 10g
- Fiber: 3g
- Sugar: 3g

Quinoa Avocado Salad

Prep Time: 15 mins

Total Time: 20 mins

Servings: 2

Ingredients:

- 1 cup cooked quinoa, cooled
- 1 avocado, diced
- 1/4 cup cherry tomatoes, halved
- 1/4 cup cucumber, diced
- 1/4 cup red onion, thinly sliced
- 2 tbsp chopped fresh cilantro
- Juice of 1 lime
- 2 tbsp olive oil
- Salt and pepper to taste
- 1 scoop collagen powder (optional)

Directions:

1. In a large bowl, combine cooked quinoa, diced avocado, halved cherry tomatoes, diced cucumber, sliced red onion, and chopped fresh cilantro.
2. In a small bowl, whisk together lime juice, olive oil, salt, pepper, and collagen powder (if using).

3. Pour the dressing over the salad mixture.

4. Toss gently to combine.

5. Serve immediately.

Nutritional Information (per serving):

- Calories: 320
- Protein: 7g
- Fat: 21g
- Carbohydrates: 30g
- Fiber: 9g
- Sugar: 3g

Greek Salad

Prep Time: 15 mins

Total Time: 15 mins

Servings: 2

Ingredients:

- 4 cups mixed greens (e.g., romaine, iceberg, spinach)
- 1/4 cup cherry tomatoes, halved
- 1/4 cup cucumber, sliced
- 1/4 cup red onion, thinly sliced
- 1/4 cup Kalamata olives
- 1/4 cup crumbled feta cheese
- Juice of 1 lemon
- 2 tbsp olive oil
- 1 tsp dried oregano
- Salt and pepper to taste
- 1 scoop collagen powder (optional)

Directions:

1. In a large bowl, combine mixed greens, halved cherry tomatoes, sliced cucumber, sliced red onion, Kalamata olives, and crumbled feta cheese.
2. In a small bowl, whisk together lemon juice, olive oil, dried oregano, salt, pepper, and collagen powder (if using).
3. Pour the dressing over the salad mixture.
4. Toss gently to combine.
5. Serve immediately.

Nutritional Information (per serving):

- Calories: 280
- Protein: 8g
- Fat: 20g
- Carbohydrates: 15g
- Fiber: 6g
- Sugar: 5g

Beet and Goat Cheese Salad

Prep Time: 20 mins

Total Time: 25 mins

Servings: 2

Ingredients:

- 4 cups mixed greens (e.g., arugula, spinach, spring mix)
- 1 large beet, roasted and diced
- 1/4 cup walnuts, chopped
- 1/4 cup goat cheese, crumbled
- 2 tbsp balsamic vinegar

- 2 tbsp olive oil
- Salt and pepper to taste
- 1 scoop collagen powder (optional)

Directions:

1. In a large bowl, combine mixed greens, roasted and diced beet, chopped walnuts, and crumbled goat cheese.
2. In a small bowl, whisk together balsamic vinegar, olive oil, salt, pepper, and collagen powder (if using).
3. Pour the dressing over the salad mixture.
4. Toss gently to combine.
5. Serve immediately.

Nutritional Information (per serving):

- Calories: 310
- Protein: 8g
- Fat: 25g
- Carbohydrates: 15g
- Fiber: 5g
- Sugar: 7g

Spinach and Strawberry Salad

Prep Time: 10 mins

Total Time: 10 mins

Servings: 2

Ingredients:

- 4 cups baby spinach
- 1 cup sliced strawberries
- 1/4 cup sliced almonds

- 1/4 cup crumbled feta cheese
- 2 tbsp balsamic vinegar
- 2 tbsp olive oil
- Salt and pepper to taste
- 1 scoop collagen powder (optional)

Directions:

1. In a large bowl, combine baby spinach, sliced strawberries, sliced almonds, and crumbled feta cheese.
2. In a small bowl, whisk together balsamic vinegar, olive oil, salt, pepper, and collagen powder (if using).
3. Drizzle the dressing over the salad mixture.
4. Toss gently to combine.
5. Serve immediately.

Nutritional Information (per serving):

- Calories: 230
- Protein: 7g
- Fat: 16g
- Carbohydrates: 17g
- Fiber: 6g
- Sugar: 7g

Mediterranean Chickpea Salad

Prep Time: 15 mins

Total Time: 15 mins

Servings: 2

Ingredients:

- 1 can (15 oz) chickpeas, drained and rinsed

- 1 cup cherry tomatoes, halved
- 1/4 cup diced cucumber
- 1/4 cup diced red onion
- 1/4 cup chopped fresh parsley
- 2 tbsp lemon juice
- 2 tbsp olive oil
- Salt and pepper to taste
- 1 scoop collagen powder (optional)

Directions:

1. In a large bowl, combine chickpeas, cherry tomatoes, diced cucumber, diced red onion, and chopped fresh parsley.
2. In a small bowl, whisk together lemon juice, olive oil, salt, pepper, and collagen powder (if using).
3. Pour the dressing over the salad mixture.
4. Toss gently to combine.
5. Serve immediately.

Nutritional Information (per serving):

- Calories: 270
- Protein: 8g
- Fat: 14g
- Carbohydrates: 29g
- Fiber: 8g
- Sugar: 6g

Asian Sesame Kale Salad

Prep Time: 15 mins

Total Time: 15 mins

Servings: 2

Ingredients:

- 4 cups chopped kale
- 1/4 cup shredded carrots
- 1/4 cup sliced red bell pepper
- 1/4 cup sliced cucumber
- 2 tbsp sesame seeds
- 2 tbsp soy sauce
- 1 tbsp rice vinegar
- 1 tbsp sesame oil
- 1 tsp honey
- 1 scoop collagen powder (optional)

Directions:

1. In a large bowl, combine chopped kale, shredded carrots, sliced red bell pepper, sliced cucumber, and sesame seeds.
2. In a small bowl, whisk together soy sauce, rice vinegar, sesame oil, honey, and collagen powder (if using).
3. Pour the dressing over the salad mixture.
4. Toss gently to combine.
5. Serve immediately.

Nutritional Information (per serving):

- Calories: 180
- Protein: 8g
- Fat: 11g
- Carbohydrates: 19g
- Fiber: 4g

- Sugar: 6g

Apple Walnut Salad

Prep Time: 10 mins

Total Time: 10 mins

Servings: 2

Ingredients:

- 4 cups mixed greens (e.g., arugula, spinach, spring mix)
- 1 apple, thinly sliced
- 1/4 cup chopped walnuts
- 1/4 cup crumbled blue cheese
- 2 tbsp apple cider vinegar
- 2 tbsp olive oil
- Salt and pepper to taste
- 1 scoop collagen powder (optional)

Directions:

1. In a large bowl, combine mixed greens, thinly sliced apple, chopped walnuts, and crumbled blue cheese.
2. In a small bowl, whisk together apple cider vinegar, olive oil, salt, pepper, and collagen powder (if using).
3. Pour the dressing over the salad mixture.
4. Toss gently to combine.
5. Serve immediately.

Nutritional Information (per serving):

- Calories: 280
- Protein: 7g
- Fat: 21g

- Carbohydrates: 18g
- Fiber: 5g
- Sugar: 11g

Caprese Salad

Prep Time: 10 mins

Total Time: 10 mins

Servings: 2

Ingredients:

- 2 large tomatoes, sliced
- 4 oz fresh mozzarella cheese, sliced
- 1/4 cup fresh basil leaves
- 2 tbsp balsamic glaze
- 2 tbsp olive oil
- Salt and pepper to taste
- 1 scoop collagen powder (optional)

Directions:

1. Arrange tomato slices and fresh mozzarella slices alternately on a serving platter.
2. Tuck fresh basil leaves between the tomato and mozzarella slices.
3. Drizzle balsamic glaze and olive oil over the salad.
4. Season with salt, pepper, and collagen powder (if using).
5. Serve immediately.

Nutritional Information (per serving):

- Calories: 290
- Protein: 12g

- Fat: 22g
- Carbohydrates: 11g
- Fiber: 2g
- Sugar: 7g

BEVERAGES RECIPES

Berry Blast Collagen Smoothie

- **Prep Time:** 5 mins
- **Total Time:** 5 mins
- **Servings:** 2 glasses

Ingredients:

- 1 cup frozen mixed berries
- 1/2 cup ice made with filtered or spring water
- 1 cup coconut water
- 1 1/2 cups spinach
- 1/2 avocado
- 1 tsp honey
- 1 scoop collagen powder
- Optional: 1 tbsp chia seeds

Directions:

1. In a blender, combine frozen mixed berries, ice, coconut water, spinach, avocado, honey, and collagen powder.
2. Blend until smooth.
3. If desired, add chia seeds and pulse until just combined.
4. Pour into glasses and serve immediately.

Nutritional Information (per serving):

- Calories: 180
- Protein: 6g
- Fat: 8g
- Carbohydrates: 25g

- Fiber: 9g

- Sugar: 12g

Tropical Collagen Smoothie

- **Prep Time:** 5 mins

- **Total Time:** 5 mins

- **Servings:** 2 glasses

Ingredients:

- 1 cup frozen pineapple chunks

- 1/2 cup ice made with filtered or spring water

- 1 cup coconut water

- 1/2 cup kale

- 1/2 banana

- 1 tbsp coconut oil

- 1 scoop collagen powder

Directions:

1. In a blender, combine frozen pineapple chunks, ice, coconut water, kale, banana, coconut oil, and collagen powder.

2. Blend until smooth.

3. Pour into glasses and serve immediately.

Nutritional Information (per serving):

- Calories: 200

- Protein: 7g

- Fat: 6g

- Carbohydrates: 30g

- Fiber: 5g

- Sugar: 18g

Green Goddess Collagen Smoothie

Prep Time: 5 mins

Total Time: 5 mins

Servings: 2 glasses

Ingredients:

- 1 cup frozen mango chunks
- 1/2 cup ice made with filtered or spring water
- 1 cup almond milk
- 1 cup spinach
- 1/2 avocado
- Juice of 1 lime
- 1 scoop collagen powder

Directions:

1. In a blender, combine frozen mango chunks, ice, almond milk, spinach, avocado, lime juice, and collagen powder.
2. Blend until smooth.
3. Pour into glasses and serve immediately.

Nutritional Information (per serving):

- Calories: 220
- Protein: 7g
- Fat: 9g
- Carbohydrates: 30g
- Fiber: 8g
- Sugar: 20g

Cocoa Banana Collagen Smoothie

Prep Time: 5 mins

Total Time: 5 mins

Servings: 2 glasses

Ingredients:

- 1 cup frozen banana slices
- 1/2 cup ice made with filtered or spring water
- 1 cup almond milk
- 2 tbsp cocoa powder
- 1 tbsp almond butter
- 1 scoop collagen powder
- Optional: 1 tsp honey or maple syrup for added sweetness

Directions:

1. In a blender, combine frozen banana slices, ice, almond milk, cocoa powder, almond butter, collagen powder, and optional sweetener.
2. Blend until smooth.
3. Pour into glasses and serve immediately.

Nutritional Information (per serving):

- Calories: 240
- Protein: 8g
- Fat: 10g
- Carbohydrates: 35g
- Fiber: 8g
- Sugar: 18g

Berry Spinach Collagen Smoothie

Prep Time: 5 mins

Total Time: 5 mins

Servings: 2 glasses

Ingredients:

- 1 cup frozen mixed berries
- 1/2 cup ice made with filtered or spring water
- 1 cup almond milk
- 2 cups spinach
- 1/2 banana
- 1 scoop collagen powder

Directions:

1. In a blender, combine frozen mixed berries, ice, almond milk, spinach, banana, and collagen powder.
2. Blend until smooth.
3. Pour into glasses and serve immediately.

Nutritional Information (per serving):

- Calories: 200
- Protein: 7g
- Fat: 5g
- Carbohydrates: 30g
- Fiber: 8g
- Sugar: 15g

Citrus Collagen Refresher

- **Prep Time:** 5 mins
- **Total Time:** 5 mins
- **Servings:** 2 glasses

Ingredients:

- 1 cup fresh orange juice

- 1/2 cup ice made with filtered or spring water
- 1/2 cup coconut water
- 1/2 cup cucumber, chopped
- 1/2 cup celery, chopped
- 1/2-inch piece of ginger, peeled
- 1 scoop collagen powder
- Optional: Mint leaves for garnish

Directions:

1. In a blender, combine fresh orange juice, ice, coconut water, cucumber, celery, ginger, and collagen powder.
2. Blend until smooth.
3. Pour into glasses and garnish with mint leaves if desired.
4. Serve immediately.

Nutritional Information (per serving):

- Calories: 90
- Protein: 5g
- Fat: 1g
- Carbohydrates: 18g
- Fiber: 2g
- Sugar: 12g

Pineapple Coconut Collagen Smoothie

Prep Time: 5 mins

Total Time: 5 mins

Servings: 2 glasses

Ingredients:

- 1 cup frozen pineapple chunks

- 1/2 cup ice made with filtered or spring water

- 1 cup coconut milk

- 1/2 banana

- 1 scoop collagen powder

- Optional: Unsweetened shredded coconut for garnish

Directions:

1. In a blender, combine frozen pineapple chunks, ice, coconut milk, banana, and collagen powder.

2. Blend until smooth.

3. Pour into glasses and garnish with shredded coconut if desired.

4. Serve immediately.

Nutritional Information (per serving):

- Calories: 180

- Protein: 7g

- Fat: 8g

- Carbohydrates: 25g

- Fiber: 3g

- Sugar: 16g

Green Tea Collagen Elixir

- **Prep Time:** 5 mins

- **Total Time:** 10 mins (including cooling time)

- **Servings:** 2 glasses

Ingredients:

- 2 green tea bags

- 2 cups hot water

- 1/2 cup ice made with filtered or spring water

- 1/2 cup almond milk

- 1 tbsp honey

- 1 scoop collagen powder

Directions:

1. Steep the green tea bags in hot water for 5 minutes. Remove the tea bags and let the tea cool to room temperature.

2. In a blender, combine the cooled green tea, ice, almond milk, honey, and collagen powder.

3. Blend until smooth.

4. Pour into glasses and serve immediately.

Nutritional Information (per serving):

- Calories: 70

- Protein: 5g

- Fat: 2g

- Carbohydrates: 10g

- Fiber: 0g

- Sugar: 9g

Berry Beet Collagen Booster

Prep Time: 10 mins

Total Time: 10 mins

Servings: 2 glasses

Ingredients:

- 1 cup mixed berries (strawberries, blueberries, raspberries)

- 1/2 cup ice made with filtered or spring water

- 1/2 cup beetroot juice

- 1/2 cup almond milk

- 1 tbsp lemon juice
- 1 scoop collagen powder

Directions:

1. In a blender, combine mixed berries, ice, beetroot juice, almond milk, lemon juice, and collagen powder.
2. Blend until smooth.
3. Pour into glasses and serve immediately.

Nutritional Information (per serving):

- Calories: 110
- Protein: 6g
- Fat: 2g
- Carbohydrates: 20g
- Fiber: 5g
- Sugar: 14g

Chocolate Peanut Butter Collagen Shake

Prep Time: 5 mins

Total Time: 5 mins

Servings: 2 glasses

Ingredients:

- 2 cups unsweetened almond milk
- 2 tbsp cocoa powder
- 2 tbsp natural peanut butter
- 1 scoop collagen powder
- 1/2 cup ice made with filtered or spring water
- Optional: Stevia or honey to taste

Directions:

1. In a blender, combine unsweetened almond milk, cocoa powder, peanut butter, collagen powder, and ice.
2. Blend until smooth.
3. Add stevia or honey to taste, if desired.
4. Pour into glasses and serve immediately.

Nutritional Information (per serving):

- Calories: 180
- Protein: 10g
- Fat: 12g
- Carbohydrates: 9g
- Fiber: 4g
- Sugar: 2g

Mango Banana Collagen Smoothie

Prep Time: 5 mins

Total Time: 5 mins

Servings: 2 glasses

Ingredients:

- 1 ripe mango, peeled and diced
- 1 ripe banana
- 1/2 cup ice made with filtered or spring water
- 1 cup coconut water
- 1 scoop collagen powder
- Optional: 1 tablespoon chia seeds

Directions:

1. In a blender, combine diced mango, banana, ice, coconut water, and collagen powder.

2. Blend until smooth.

3. Optionally, stir in chia seeds for added fiber and omega-3s.

4. Pour into glasses and serve immediately.

Nutritional Information (per serving):

- Calories: 180

- Protein: 7g

- Fat: 1g

- Carbohydrates: 40g

- Fiber: 5g

- Sugar: 30g

Berry Spinach Collagen Booster

Prep Time: 5 mins

Total Time: 5 mins

Servings: 2 glasses

Ingredients:

- 1 cup mixed berries (strawberries, blueberries, raspberries)

- 1 handful spinach leaves

- 1/2 cup ice made with filtered or spring water

- 1 cup almond milk

- 1 scoop collagen powder

- Optional: 1 tablespoon honey for sweetness

Directions:

1. In a blender, combine mixed berries, spinach leaves, ice, almond milk, and collagen powder.

2. Blend until smooth.

3. Optionally, add honey for sweetness if desired.

4. Pour into glasses and serve immediately.

Nutritional Information (per serving):

- Calories: 140
- Protein: 7g
- Fat: 3g
- Carbohydrates: 25g
- Fiber: 6g
- Sugar: 16g

Turmeric Ginger Collagen Elixir

Prep Time: 5 mins

Total Time: 10 mins (including cooling time)

Servings: 2 glasses

Ingredients:

- 2 cups almond milk
- 1/2 teaspoon ground turmeric
- 1/2 teaspoon ground ginger
- 1/2 teaspoon cinnamon
- 1 scoop collagen powder
- Optional: 1 tablespoon honey for sweetness

Directions:

1. In a small saucepan, heat almond milk over low heat.
2. Whisk in ground turmeric, ginger, and cinnamon until fully combined. Let it simmer for 5 minutes.
3. Remove from heat and let it cool slightly.
4. In a blender, combine the spiced almond milk with collagen powder.

5. Blend until smooth.

6. Optionally, add honey for sweetness if desired.

7. Pour into glasses and serve warm.

Nutritional Information (per serving):

- Calories: 120

- Protein: 6g

- Fat: 4g

- Carbohydrates: 15g

- Fiber: 1g

- Sugar: 10g

Avocado Matcha Collagen Latte

Ingredients:

- 1 ripe avocado

- 1 teaspoon matcha powder

- 1 cup almond milk

- 1 scoop collagen powder

- Optional: 1 tablespoon maple syrup for sweetness

Directions:

1. In a blender, combine ripe avocado, matcha powder, almond milk, and collagen powder.

2. Blend until smooth.

3. Optionally, add maple syrup for sweetness if desired.

4. Pour into glasses and serve immediately.

Nutritional Information (per serving):

- Calories: 150

- Protein: 6g

- Fat: 9g
- Carbohydrates: 10g
- Fiber: 5
- Sugar: 3g

Pineapple Cucumber Collagen Cooler

Prep Time: 5 mins

Total Time: 5 mins

Servings: 2 glasses

Ingredients:

- 1 cup fresh pineapple chunks
- 1/2 cucumber, peeled and chopped
- 1/2 cup ice made with filtered or spring water
- 1 cup coconut water
- 1 scoop collagen powder
- Optional: Fresh mint leaves for garnish

Directions:

1. In a blender, combine fresh pineapple chunks, chopped cucumber, ice, coconut water, and collagen powder.
2. Blend until smooth.
3. Pour into glasses and garnish with fresh mint leaves if desired.
4. Serve immediately.

Nutritional Information (per serving):

- Calories: 120
- Protein: 5g
- Fat: 1g
- Carbohydrates: 25g

- Fiber: 3g
- Sugar: 18g

Matcha Green Tea Collagen Latte

Prep Time: 5 mins

Total Time: 5 mins

Servings: 2 glasses

Ingredients:

- 2 tsp matcha green tea powder
- 1 cup hot water
- 1/2 cup coconut milk
- 1 scoop collagen powder
- 1 tsp honey or maple syrup (optional)

Directions:

1. In a small bowl, whisk together matcha green tea powder and hot water until dissolved.
2. In a saucepan, heat coconut milk until warm but not boiling.
3. Pour the warm coconut milk into a blender, add the dissolved matcha green tea, collagen powder, and honey or maple syrup if using.
4. Blend until smooth and frothy.
5. Pour into glasses and serve immediately.

Nutritional Information (per serving):

- Calories: 90
- Protein: 7g
- Fat: 4g
- Carbohydrates: 8g

- Fiber: 1g

- Sugar: 5g

Berry Collagen Smoothie Bowl

Prep Time: 5 mins

Total Time: 5 mins

Servings: 2 bowls

Ingredients:

- 1 cup frozen mixed berries

- 1/2 cup unsweetened almond milk

- 1 scoop collagen powder

- 1/2 banana, sliced

- 1/4 cup granola

- Optional toppings: sliced almonds, chia seeds, shredded coconut

Directions:

1. In a blender, combine frozen mixed berries, almond milk, and collagen powder.
2. Blend until smooth and creamy.
3. Pour the smoothie into bowls.
4. Top with sliced banana, granola, and any additional toppings as desired.
5. Serve immediately.

Nutritional Information (per serving):

- Calories: 180

- Protein: 10g

- Fat: 5g

- Carbohydrates: 25g

- Fiber: 5g

- Sugar: 10g

Tropical Collagen Refresher

Prep Time: 5 mins

Total Time: 5 mins

Servings: 2 glasses

Ingredients:

- 1/2 cup pineapple chunks

- 1/2 cup mango chunks

- 1/2 cup coconut water

- 1/2 cup unsweetened almond milk

- 1 scoop collagen powder

- 1/2 cup ice cubes

Directions:

1. In a blender, combine pineapple chunks, mango chunks, coconut water, almond milk, collagen powder, and ice cubes.

2. Blend until smooth.

3. Pour into glasses and serve immediately.

Nutritional Information (per serving):

- Calories: 120

- Protein: 6g

- Fat: 3g

- Carbohydrates: 20g

- Fiber: 3g

- Sugar: 15g

Cucumber Mint Collagen Cooler

Prep Time: 5 mins

Total Time: 5 mins

Servings: 2 glasses

Ingredients:

- 1 cucumber, peeled and chopped
- 1/4 cup fresh mint leaves
- 1 cup coconut water
- 1/2 cup ice cubes
- 1 scoop collagen powder
- 1 tsp honey (optional)

Directions:

1. In a blender, combine chopped cucumber, fresh mint leaves, coconut water, ice cubes, collagen powder, and honey if using.
2. Blend until smooth.
3. Pour into glasses and serve immediately.

Nutritional Information (per serving):

- Calories: 70
- Protein: 5g
- Fat: 1g
- Carbohydrates: 15g
- Fiber: 2g
- Sugar: 10g

Golden Turmeric Collagen Elixir

Prep Time: 5 mins

Total Time: 5 mins

Servings: 2 glasses

Ingredients:

- 1 cup unsweetened almond milk
- 1/2 tsp ground turmeric
- 1/4 tsp ground cinnamon
- Pinch of ground black pepper
- 1 scoop collagen powder
- 1/2 tsp honey or maple syrup (optional)

Directions:

1. In a saucepan, heat almond milk over medium heat until warm but not boiling.
2. Stir in ground turmeric, ground cinnamon, ground black pepper, collagen powder, and honey or maple syrup if using.
3. Whisk until well combined and heated through.
4. Pour into glasses and serve immediately.

Nutritional Information (per serving):

- Calories: 80
- Protein: 7g
- Fat: 3g
- Carbohydras

DESSERTS RECIPES

Coconut Chia Pudding

Prep Time: 5 minutes

Total Time: 4 hours 5 minutes

Servings: 2

Ingredients:

- 1/4 cup chia seeds
- 1 cup coconut milk
- 1 teaspoon vanilla extract
- 1 tablespoon honey or maple syrup
- Sliced strawberries or other fresh fruits for topping

Directions:

1. In a bowl, mix chia seeds, coconut milk, vanilla extract, and sweetener.
2. Cover and refrigerate for at least 4 hours, preferably overnight, until it reaches a pudding-like consistency.
3. Stir well before serving, and top with sliced strawberries or your favorite fruits.

Nutritional Information (per serving):

- Calories: 236
- Protein: 4g
- Fat: 18g
- Carbohydrates: 17g
- Fiber: 10g
- Sugar: 5g

Avocado Chocolate Mousse

Prep Time: 10 minutes

Total Time: 10 minutes

Servings: 2

Ingredients:

- 1 ripe avocado
- 3 tablespoons cocoa powder
- 2 tablespoons honey or maple syrup
- 1/2 teaspoon vanilla extract
- Pinch of salt
- Fresh berries for garnish

Directions:

1. Scoop the flesh of the avocado into a blender or food processor.
2. Add cocoa powder, honey or maple syrup, vanilla extract, and a pinch of salt.
3. Blend until smooth and creamy.
4. Divide into serving dishes and refrigerate for at least 30 minutes.
5. Serve chilled, garnished with fresh berries.

Nutritional Information (per serving):

- Calories: 220
- Protein: 3g
- Fat: 14g
- Carbohydrates: 27g
- Fiber: 8g
- Sugar: 15g

Berry Collagen Gelatin

Prep Time: 5 minutes

Total Time: 3 hours 5 minutes

Servings: 4

Ingredients:

- 1 cup mixed berries (strawberries, blueberries, raspberries)
- 2 tablespoons grass-fed gelatin powder
- 1 cup water
- 1 tablespoon honey or maple syrup (optional)
- 1 scoop collagen powder

Directions:

1. In a saucepan, combine water and gelatin powder. Let it sit for a few minutes to bloom.
2. Heat the mixture over low heat, stirring until the gelatin dissolves completely.
3. Remove from heat and stir in honey or maple syrup if using.
4. Add the berries to a bowl or individual serving dishes.
5. Pour the gelatin mixture over the berries.
6. Refrigerate for at least 3 hours, or until set.
7. Serve chilled.

Nutritional Information (per serving):

- Calories: 60
- Protein: 7g
- Fat: 0g
- Carbohydrates: 6g
- Fiber: 1g

- Sugar: 4g

Coconut Collagen Popsicles

Prep Time: 10 minutes

Total Time: 4 hours 10 minutes

Servings: 4

Ingredients:

- 1 cup coconut milk
- 1/4 cup shredded coconut
- 1 tablespoon honey or maple syrup
- 1 teaspoon vanilla extract
- 1 scoop collagen powder

Directions:

1. In a blender, combine coconut milk, shredded coconut, honey or maple syrup, vanilla extract, and collagen powder. Blend until smooth.
2. Pour the mixture into popsicle molds.
3. Insert popsicle sticks and freeze for at least 4 hours, or until completely frozen.
4. Remove from molds and enjoy.

Nutritional Information (per serving):

- Calories: 105
- Protein: 3g
- Fat: 9g
- Carbohydrates: 6g
- Fiber: 1g
- Sugar: 4g

Vanilla Collagen Custard

Prep Time: 5 minutes

Total Time: 25 minutes

Servings: 2

Ingredients:

- 2 cups coconut milk
- 2 tablespoons honey or maple syrup
- 1 teaspoon vanilla extract
- 2 tablespoons grass-fed gelatin powder
- 1 scoop collagen powder

Directions:

1. In a saucepan, heat coconut milk over medium heat until warm but not boiling.
2. Stir in honey or maple syrup and vanilla extract until dissolved.
3. Gradually whisk in the gelatin powder until fully dissolved.
4. Remove from heat and stir in the collagen powder until smooth.
5. Pour into serving dishes and refrigerate for at least 2 hours, or until set.
6. Serve chilled.

Nutritional Information (per serving):

- Calories: 300
- Protein: 9g
- Fat: 21g
- Carbohydrates: 19g
- Fiber: 0g
- Sugar: 14g

Blueberry Collagen Parfait

Prep Time: 10 mins

Total Time: 10 mins

Servings: 2

Ingredients:

- 1 cup frozen organic blueberries
- 1/2 cup Greek yogurt
- 2 tablespoons honey
- 1 scoop collagen powder
- 1/4 cup granola
- Fresh mint leaves for garnish (optional)

Directions:

1. In a bowl, mix Greek yogurt, honey, and collagen powder until well combined.
2. In serving glasses, layer the yogurt mixture with frozen blueberries and granola.
3. Repeat the layers until the glasses are filled.
4. Garnish with fresh mint leaves if desired.
5. Serve immediately.

Nutritional Information (per serving):

- Calories: 280
- Protein: 16g
- Fat: 5g
- Carbohydrates: 45g
- Fiber: 5g
- Sugar: 28g

Coconut Collagen Balls

Prep Time: 15 mins

Total Time: 1 hour 15 mins

Servings: 10 balls

Ingredients:

- 1 cup shredded coconut
- 1/4 cup coconut flour
- 2 tablespoons honey
- 2 tablespoons coconut oil, melted
- 1 scoop collagen powder
- 1 teaspoon vanilla extract
- Pinch of salt

Directions:

1. In a bowl, mix shredded coconut, coconut flour, honey, melted coconut oil, collagen powder, vanilla extract, and a pinch of salt until well combined.
2. Roll the mixture into small balls and place them on a baking sheet lined with parchment paper.
3. Refrigerate for at least 1 hour, or until firm.
4. Serve chilled.

Nutritional Information (per serving - 1 ball):

- Calories: 120
- Protein: 2g
- Fat: 9g
- Carbohydrates: 8g
- Fiber: 3g

- Sugar: 4g

Chocolate Collagen Pudding

Prep Time: 5 mins

Total Time: 2 hours 5 mins

Servings: 2

Ingredients:

- 1 ripe avocado
- 3 tablespoons cocoa powder
- 2 tablespoons honey or maple syrup
- 1 scoop collagen powder
- 1/2 teaspoon vanilla extract
- Pinch of salt

Directions:

1. Scoop the flesh of the avocado into a blender or food processor.
2. Add cocoa powder, honey or maple syrup, collagen powder, vanilla extract, and a pinch of salt.
3. Blend until smooth and creamy.
4. Divide into serving dishes and refrigerate for at least 2 hours, or until set.
5. Serve chilled.

Nutritional Information (per serving):

- Calories: 280
- Protein: 7g
- Fat: 19g
- Carbohydrates: 30g
- Fiber: 9g

- Sugar: 17g

Fruit Salad with Collagen-Infused Dressing

Prep Time: 10 mins

Total Time: 10 mins

Servings: 2

Ingredients:

- 1 cup mixed fresh fruits (such as strawberries, kiwi, mango, and pineapple)
- 1 tablespoon lemon juice
- 1 tablespoon honey
- 1 scoop collagen powder

Directions:

1. In a bowl, combine mixed fresh fruits.
2. In a small bowl, whisk together lemon juice, honey, and collagen powder until smooth.
3. Drizzle the dressing over the fruit salad and toss gently to coat.
4. Serve immediately.

Nutritional Information (per serving):

- Calories: 120
- Protein: 2g
- Fat: 0g
- Carbohydrates: 30g
- Fiber: 4g
- Sugar: 24g

Vanilla Collagen Rice Pudding

Prep Time: 5 mins

Total Time: 25 mins

Servings: 2

Ingredients:

- 1/2 cup cooked white rice
- 1 cup coconut milk
- 2 tablespoons honey or maple syrup
- 1 scoop collagen powder
- 1 teaspoon vanilla extract
- Pinch of cinnamon (optional)

Directions:

1. In a saucepan, combine cooked white rice, coconut milk, honey or maple syrup, collagen powder, vanilla extract, and a pinch of cinnamon if using.
2. Cook over medium heat, stirring occasionally, until the mixture thickens and reaches a pudding-like consistency, about 20 minutes.
3. Remove from heat and let it cool slightly.
4. Divide into serving dishes and serve warm or chilled.

Nutritional Information (per serving):

- Calories: 250
- Protein: 6g
- Fat: 8g
- Carbohydrates: 40g
- Fiber: 1g
- Sugar: 18g

Chia Seed Pudding with Berries

Prep Time: 5 mins

Total Time: 4 hours 5 mins

Servings: 2

Ingredients:

- 1/4 cup chia seeds
- 1 cup coconut milk
- 1 tablespoon honey or maple syrup
- 1 scoop collagen powder
- 1/2 teaspoon vanilla extract
- Fresh berries for topping

Directions:

1. In a bowl, mix chia seeds, coconut milk, honey or maple syrup, collagen powder, and vanilla extract.
2. Cover and refrigerate for at least 4 hours or overnight, until the mixture thickens and sets.
3. Stir the pudding well before serving.
4. Divide into serving bowls and top with fresh berries.
5. Serve chilled.

Nutritional Information (per serving):

- Calories: 250
- Protein: 8g
- Fat: 16g
- Carbohydrates: 22g
- Fiber: 10g
- Sugar: 7g

Collagen-Infused Mango Sorbet

Prep Time: 10 mins

Total Time: 3 hours 10 mins

Servings: 2

Ingredients:

- 2 ripe mangoes, peeled and diced
- 2 tablespoons honey or maple syrup
- 1 scoop collagen powder
- Juice of 1 lime
- Fresh mint leaves for garnish (optional)

Directions:

1. Place diced mangoes in a blender or food processor.
2. Add honey or maple syrup, collagen powder, and lime juice.
3. Blend until smooth.
4. Transfer the mixture into a shallow dish and freeze for about 3 hours, stirring every 30 minutes until it reaches a sorbet consistency.
5. Serve in bowls, garnished with fresh mint leaves if desired.

Nutritional Information (per serving):

- Calories: 180
- Protein: 5g
- Fat: 1g
- Carbohydrates: 45g
- Fiber: 5g
- Sugar: 37g

Coconut Collagen Bliss Balls

- **Prep Time:** 15 mins
- **Total Time:** 15 mins
- **Servings:** 10 balls

Ingredients:

- 1 cup shredded coconut
- 1/4 cup almond flour
- 2 tablespoons honey or maple syrup
- 1 scoop collagen powder
- 2 tablespoons coconut oil, melted
- 1 teaspoon vanilla extract
- Pinch of salt

Directions:

1. In a bowl, mix shredded coconut, almond flour, honey or maple syrup, collagen powder, melted coconut oil, vanilla extract, and a pinch of salt until well combined.
2. Roll the mixture into small balls.
3. Refrigerate for at least 30 minutes before serving.
4. Serve chilled.

Nutritional Information (per serving - 1 ball):

- Calories: 120
- Protein: 2g
- Fat: 10g
- Carbohydrates: 7g
- Fiber: 3g
- Sugar: 4g

Collagen-Infused Banana Ice Cream

Prep Time: 5 mins

Total Time: 3 hours 5 mins

Servings: 2

Ingredients:

- 2 ripe bananas, sliced and frozen
- 2 tablespoons almond butter
- 1 scoop collagen powder
- 1/2 teaspoon vanilla extract
- Pinch of cinnamon (optional)

Directions:

1. Place frozen banana slices, almond butter, collagen powder, vanilla extract, and cinnamon if using in a blender or food processor.
2. Blend until smooth and creamy.
3. Transfer the mixture into a shallow dish and freeze for about 3 hours, stirring every 30 minutes until it reaches a creamy ice cream consistency.
4. Serve in bowls.

Nutritional Information (per serving):

- Calories: 200
- Protein: 6g
- Fat: 6g
- Carbohydrates: 35g
- Fiber: 5g
- Sugar: 17g

Chocolate Collagen Avocado Mousse

Prep Time: 10 mins

Total Time: 2 hours 10 mins

Servings: 2

Ingredients:

- 1 ripe avocado
- 3 tablespoons cocoa powder
- 2 tablespoons honey or maple syrup
- 1 scoop collagen powder
- 1/2 teaspoon vanilla extract
- Pinch of salt

Directions:

1. Scoop the flesh of the avocado into a blender or food processor.
2. Add cocoa powder, honey or maple syrup, collagen powder, vanilla extract, and a pinch of salt.
3. Blend until smooth and creamy.
4. Divide into serving dishes and refrigerate for at least 2 hours, or until set.
5. Serve chilled.

Nutritional Information (per serving):

- Calories: 280
- Protein: 7g
- Fat: 19g
- Carbohydrates: 30g
- Fiber: 9g
- Sugar: 17g

Coconut Collagen Popsicles

Prep Time: 10 mins

Total Time: 6 hours 10 mins

Servings: 6 popsicles

Ingredients:

- 1 cup coconut milk
- 1/4 cup shredded coconut
- 2 tablespoons honey or maple syrup
- 1 scoop collagen powder
- 1 teaspoon vanilla extract
- Pinch of salt

Directions:

1. In a blender, combine coconut milk, shredded coconut, honey or maple syrup, collagen powder, vanilla extract, and a pinch of salt.
2. Blend until smooth.
3. Pour the mixture into popsicle molds.
4. Insert popsicle sticks into each mold.
5. Freeze for at least 6 hours or until solid.
6. To remove the popsicles from the molds, run warm water over the outside of the mold for a few seconds.
7. Serve immediately.

Nutritional Information (per serving):

- Calories: 120
- Protein: 3g
- Fat: 9g
- Carbohydrates: 9g

- Fiber: 1g

- Sugar: 7g

Berry Collagen Chia Pudding

Prep Time: 5 mins

Total Time: 4 hours 5 mins

Servings: 2

Ingredients:

- 1 cup mixed berries (such as strawberries, blueberries, raspberries)

- 1 cup coconut milk

- 2 tablespoons honey or maple syrup

- 2 tablespoons chia seeds

- 1 scoop collagen powder

- 1/2 teaspoon vanilla extract

Directions:

1. In a blender, combine mixed berries, coconut milk, honey or maple syrup, collagen powder, and vanilla extract.

2. Blend until smooth.

3. Transfer the mixture to a bowl and stir in chia seeds.

4. Cover and refrigerate for at least 4 hours or overnight, until the chia seeds have absorbed the liquid and the mixture has thickened.

5. Stir well before serving.

6. Divide into serving dishes and garnish with additional berries if desired.

Nutritional Information (per serving):

- Calories: 220

- Protein: 6g

- Fat: 12g

- Carbohydrates: 24g

- Fiber: 8g

- Sugar: 13g

Chocolate Collagen Mousse

Prep Time: 15 mins

Total Time: 2 hours 15 mins

Servings: 4

Ingredients:

- 1 ripe avocado

- 1/4 cup cocoa powder

- 1/4 cup honey or maple syrup

- 1/4 cup coconut milk

- 1 scoop collagen powder

- 1 teaspoon vanilla extract

- Pinch of salt

Directions:

1. Scoop the flesh of the avocado into a blender or food processor.

2. Add cocoa powder, honey or maple syrup, coconut milk, collagen powder, vanilla extract, and a pinch of salt.

3. Blend until smooth and creamy.

4. Transfer the mousse to serving dishes.

5. Cover and refrigerate for at least 2 hours, or until set.

6. Serve chilled, garnished with shaved chocolate or berries if desired.

Nutritional Information (per serving):

- Calories: 180
- Protein: 4g
- Fat: 10g
- Carbohydrates: 23g
- Fiber: 5g
- Sugar: 16g

Vanilla Collagen Yogurt Parfait

Prep Time: 10 mins

Total Time: 10 mins

Servings: 2

Ingredients:

- 1 cup Greek yogurt
- 2 tablespoons honey or maple syrup
- 1 scoop collagen powder
- 1/2 teaspoon vanilla extract
- 1/4 cup granola
- Fresh berries for garnish (optional)

Directions:

1. In a bowl, mix Greek yogurt, honey or maple syrup, collagen powder, and vanilla extract until well combined.
2. In serving glasses, layer the yogurt mixture with granola.
3. Repeat the layers until the glasses are filled.
4. Garnish with fresh berries if desired.

5. Serve immediately.

Nutritional Information (per serving):

- Calories: 220
- Protein: 14g
- Fat: 6g
- Carbohydrates: 30g
- Fiber: 2g
- Sugar: 22g

Matcha Collagen Smoothie Bowl

Prep Time: 10 mins

Total Time: 10 mins

Servings: 2

Ingredients:

- 2 ripe bananas, sliced and frozen
- 1/2 cup coconut milk
- 1 tablespoon honey or maple syrup
- 1 teaspoon matcha powder
- 1 scoop collagen powder
- Toppings: sliced fruits, shredded coconut, chia seeds, nuts

Directions:

1. In a blender, combine frozen banana slices, coconut milk, honey or maple syrup, matcha powder, and collagen powder.
2. Blend until smooth and creamy.
3. Pour the smoothie into serving bowls.
4. Top with sliced fruits, shredded coconut, chia seeds, and nuts.
5. Serve immediately.

Nutritional Information (per serving):

- Calories: 220

- Protein

DRINKS RECIPES

Collagen Boost Smoothie

Prep Time: 5 mins

Total Time: 5 mins

Servings: 2 glasses

Ingredients:

- 1 cup frozen organic blueberries
- 1/2 cup ice made with filtered or spring water
- 1 cup coconut water or almond milk
- 1 1/2 cups mixed greens (kale, spinach, celery)
- 1/2 avocado
- 1 scoop collagen powder
- 1 tsp honey or maple syrup (optional)
- Optional additions: turmeric, chia seeds, probiotic powder

Directions:

1. In a blender, combine frozen blueberries, ice, coconut water or almond milk, mixed greens, avocado, collagen powder, and honey or maple syrup if desired.
2. Blend until smooth and creamy, adding more liquid if necessary for desired consistency.
3. Optionally, add any suggested additions like turmeric, chia seeds, or probiotic powder.
4. Pour into glasses and serve immediately.

Nutritional Information (per serving):

- Calories: 190

- Protein: 8g

- Fat: 8g

- Carbohydrates: 25g

- Fiber: 7g

- Sugar: 13g

Matcha Collagen Latte

Prep Time: 5 mins

Total Time: 5 mins

Servings: 1

Ingredients:

- 1 tsp matcha powder

- 1 cup hot water

- 1/2 cup coconut milk

- 1 scoop collagen powder

- 1 tsp honey or maple syrup (optional)

Directions:

1. In a cup, whisk matcha powder with hot water until dissolved.

2. In a small saucepan, heat coconut milk until warm but not boiling.

3. Pour the warm coconut milk into the matcha mixture.

4. Stir in collagen powder and honey or maple syrup if desired.

5. Mix well until everything is well combined and frothy.

6. Pour into a mug and serve hot.

Nutritional Information (per serving):

- Calories: 110

- Protein: 8g

- Fat: 5g

- Carbohydrates: 10g

- Fiber: 0g

- Sugar: 6g

Berry Collagen Spritzer

Prep Time: 5 mins

Total Time: 5 mins

Servings: 2

Ingredients:

- 1/2 cup mixed berries (strawberries, blueberries, raspberries)

- 1 cup sparkling water

- 1 scoop collagen powder

- Ice cubes

- Fresh mint leaves for garnish (optional)

Directions:

1. In a blender, combine mixed berries and sparkling water.

2. Blend until smooth.

3. Pour the berry mixture into glasses filled with ice cubes.

4. Stir in collagen powder until well combined.

5. Garnish with fresh mint leaves if desired.

6. Serve immediately.

Nutritional Information (per serving):

- Calories: 20

- Protein: 4g

- Fat: 0g

- Carbohydrates: 5g

- Fiber: 1g

- Sugar: 3g

Collagen Iced Coffee

Prep Time: 5 mins

Total Time: 5 mins

Servings: 1

Ingredients:

- 1 cup brewed coffee, cooled

- 1/2 cup almond milk

- 1 scoop collagen powder

- 1 tsp honey or maple syrup (optional)

- Ice cubes

Directions:

1. In a glass, combine cooled brewed coffee and almond milk.

2. Stir in collagen powder and honey or maple syrup if desired.

3. Fill the glass with ice cubes.

4. Stir well until everything is well combined.

5. Serve immediately.

Nutritional Information (per serving):

- Calories: 60

- Protein: 6g

- Fat: 2g

- Carbohydrates: 8g

- Fiber: 1g

- Sugar: 5g

Tropical Collagen Smoothie

Prep Time: 5 mins

Total Time: 5 mins

Servings: 2 glasses

Ingredients:

- 1 cup frozen mango chunks
- 1/2 cup frozen pineapple chunks
- 1 cup coconut water
- 1 scoop collagen powder
- 1/2 banana
- Juice of 1/2 lime
- Optional: shredded coconut for garnish

Directions:

1. In a blender, combine frozen mango chunks, frozen pineapple chunks, coconut water, collagen powder, banana, and lime juice.
2. Blend until smooth and creamy.
3. Pour into glasses and garnish with shredded coconut if desired.
4. Serve immediately.

Nutritional Information (per serving):

- Calories: 150
- Protein: 7g
- Fat: 1g
- Carbohydrates: 30g
- Fiber: 4

Green Collagen Smoothie

Prep Time: 5 mins

Total Time: 5 mins

Servings: 2 glasses

Ingredients:

- 1 cup frozen organic blueberries or other berries
- 1/2 cup ice made with filtered or spring water
- 1 cup coconut water or almond milk
- 1 1/2 cups mixed greens (kale, spinach, celery)
- 1/2 avocado or 1/4 cup nuts/seeds or 1 tbsp. coconut/olive oil
- 1 tsp sweetener such as honey or maple syrup (optional)
- Optional additions: turmeric, collagen powder, probiotic powder

Directions:

1. In a blender, combine frozen berries, ice, coconut water or almond milk, mixed greens, avocado or nuts/seeds/oil, and sweetener if using.
2. Add optional additions like turmeric, collagen powder, or probiotic powder for extra benefits.
3. Blend until smooth and creamy, adding more liquid if necessary for desired consistency.
4. Pour into glasses and serve immediately.

Nutritional Information (per serving):

- Calories: 220
- Protein: 5g
- Fat: 12g
- Carbohydrates: 25g

- Fiber: 10g

- Sugar: 12g

Turmeric Collagen Latte

Prep Time: 2 mins

Total Time: 7 mins

Servings: 1

Ingredients:

- 1 cup almond milk or coconut milk

- 1 tsp turmeric powder

- 1 scoop collagen powder

- 1 tsp honey or maple syrup (optional)

- Pinch of black pepper

Directions:

1. In a saucepan, heat almond milk or coconut milk over medium heat until warm but not boiling.

2. Whisk in turmeric powder, collagen powder, honey or maple syrup if using, and a pinch of black pepper.

3. Continue to heat for 2-3 minutes, stirring occasionally, until the mixture is well combined and heated through.

4. Pour into a mug and serve hot.

Nutritional Information (per serving):

- Calories: 120

- Protein: 9g

- Fat: 5g

- Carbohydrates: 15g

- Fiber: 3g

- Sugar: 10g

Berry Collagen Smoothie Bowl

Prep Time: 5 mins

Total Time: 5 mins

Servings: 1 bowl

Ingredients:

- 1 cup frozen mixed berries
- 1/2 cup coconut water or almond milk
- 1 scoop collagen powder
- 1/2 banana
- 1 tbsp chia seeds
- Toppings: sliced fruits, shredded coconut, granola

Directions:

1. In a blender, combine frozen mixed berries, coconut water or almond milk, collagen powder, banana, and chia seeds.
2. Blend until smooth and creamy.
3. Pour the smoothie into a bowl.
4. Top with sliced fruits, shredded coconut, and granola.
5. Serve immediately.

Nutritional Information (per serving):

- Calories: 300
- Protein: 12g
- Fat: 8g
- Carbohydrates: 45g
- Fiber: 10g
- Sugar: 25g

Pineapple Collagen Refresher

Prep Time: 5 mins

Total Time: 5 mins

Servings: 2 glasses

Ingredients:

- 1 cup fresh pineapple chunks
- 1/2 cup coconut water
- Juice of 1 lime
- 1 scoop collagen powder
- 1 tsp honey or maple syrup (optional)
- Ice cubes

Directions:

1. In a blender, combine fresh pineapple chunks, coconut water, lime juice, collagen powder, and honey or maple syrup if using.
2. Blend until smooth.
3. Fill glasses with ice cubes.
4. Pour the pineapple mixture over the ice.
5. Stir well and serve immediately.

Nutritional Information (per serving):

- Calories: 120
- Protein: 6g
- Fat: 1g
- Carbohydrates: 25g
- Fiber: 3g
- Sugar: 20g

Coconut Collagen Frappuccino

Prep Time: 5 mins

Total Time: 5 mins

Servings: 1

Ingredients:

- 1 cup brewed coffee, cooled
- 1/2 cup coconut milk
- 1 scoop collagen powder
- 1 tsp honey or maple syrup (optional)
- Ice cubes

Directions:

1. In a blender, combine cooled brewed coffee, coconut milk, collagen powder, and honey or maple syrup if using.
2. Add ice cubes to the blender.
3. Blend until smooth and frothy.
4. Pour into a glass and serve immediately.

Nutritional Information (per serving):

- Calories: 110
- Protein: 5g
- Fat: 8g
- Carbohydrates: 7g
- Fiber: 0g
- Sugar: 4g

Green Goddess Smoothie

Prep Time: 5 mins

Total Time: 5 mins

Servings: 2 glasses

Ingredients:

- 1 cup frozen organic mixed berries
- 1/2 cup ice made with filtered or spring water
- 1 cup coconut water
- 1 1/2 cups mixed greens (spinach, kale, chard)
- 1/2 avocado
- 1 tbsp chia seeds
- 1 tsp honey or maple syrup (optional)
- Optional additions: collagen powder, spirulina, flaxseed

Directions:

1. Place frozen mixed berries, ice, coconut water, mixed greens, avocado, and chia seeds in a blender.
2. Add honey or maple syrup if desired, along with any optional additions like collagen powder, spirulina, or flaxseed.
3. Blend on high until smooth and creamy, adding more water if needed to reach desired consistency.
4. Pour into glasses and serve immediately.

Nutritional Information (per serving):

- Calories: 220
- Protein: 5g
- Fat: 10g
- Carbohydrates: 25g
- Fiber: 10g
- Sugar: 12g

Tropical Collagen Cooler

Prep Time: 5 mins

Total Time: 5 mins

Servings: 2 glasses

Ingredients:

- 1 cup frozen pineapple chunks
- 1/2 cup ice made with filtered or spring water
- 1 cup coconut water
- 1/2 cup plain Greek yogurt
- 1 scoop collagen powder
- 1 tsp honey or maple syrup (optional)
- Juice of 1 lime

Directions:

1. Combine frozen pineapple chunks, ice, coconut water, Greek yogurt, collagen powder, honey or maple syrup (if using), and lime juice in a blender.
2. Blend until smooth and creamy.
3. Taste and adjust sweetness if necessary by adding more honey or maple syrup.
4. Pour into glasses and serve immediately.

Nutritional Information (per serving):

- Calories: 180
- Protein: 10g
- Fat: 2g
- Carbohydrates: 30g
- Fiber: 3g
- Sugar: 20g

Berry Blast Collagen Smoothie

Prep Time: 5 mins

Total Time: 5 mins

Servings: 2 glasses

Ingredients:

- 1 cup frozen mixed berries
- 1/2 cup ice made with filtered or spring water
- 1 cup almond milk
- 1 scoop collagen powder
- 1/2 banana
- 1 tbsp almond butter
- 1 tsp honey or maple syrup (optional)

Directions:

1. Blend frozen mixed berries, ice, almond milk, collagen powder, banana, almond butter, and honey or maple syrup until smooth.
2. Add more almond milk if needed to reach desired consistency.
3. Taste and adjust sweetness if necessary.
4. Pour into glasses and serve immediately.

Nutritional Information (per serving):

- Calories: 250
- Protein: 12g
- Fat: 10g
- Carbohydrates: 30g
- Fiber: 8g
- Sugar: 16g

Citrus Collagen Refresher

Prep Time: 5 mins

Total Time: 5 mins

Servings: 2 glasses

Ingredients:

- 1 cup mixed citrus fruits (orange, grapefruit, lemon)
- 1/2 cup ice made with filtered or spring water
- 1 cup coconut water
- 1 scoop collagen powder
- 1 tbsp fresh mint leaves
- 1 tsp honey or maple syrup (optional)

Directions:

1. Blend mixed citrus fruits, ice, coconut water, collagen powder, mint leaves, and honey or maple syrup until smooth.
2. Adjust sweetness to taste.
3. Pour into glasses and serve immediately.

Nutritional Information (per serving):

- Calories: 150
- Protein: 6g
- Fat: 1g
- Carbohydrates: 30g
- Fiber: 6g
- Sugar: 20g

Creamy Mango Collagen Smoothie

Prep Time: 5 mins

Total Time: 5 mins

Servings: 2 glasses

Ingredients:

- 1 cup frozen mango chunks
- 1/2 cup ice made with filtered or spring water
- 1 cup unsweetened coconut milk
- 1 scoop collagen powder
- 1/2 cup plain Greek yogurt
- 1 tsp honey or maple syrup (optional)
- Pinch of ground cinnamon

Directions:

1. Blend frozen mango chunks, ice, coconut milk, collagen powder, Greek yogurt, honey or maple syrup, and cinnamon until smooth.
2. Adjust sweetness to taste.
3. Pour into glasses and serve immediately.

Nutritional Information (per serving):

- Calories: 220
- Protein: 10g
- Fat: 5g
- Carbohydrates: 30g

Tropical Collagen Smoothie

Prep Time: 5 mins

Total Time: 5 mins

Servings: 2 glasses

Ingredients:

- 1 cup frozen pineapple chunks
- 1/2 cup ice made with filtered or spring water
- 1 cup coconut water

- 1 banana
- 1 scoop collagen powder
- 1/2 cup Greek yogurt
- 1 tbsp honey (optional)
- Optional additions: spinach, flaxseed, chia seeds

Directions:

1. In a blender, combine frozen pineapple chunks, ice, coconut water, banana, collagen powder, Greek yogurt, and honey.
2. Add any optional additions like spinach, flaxseed, or chia seeds if desired.
3. Blend until smooth and creamy.
4. Pour into glasses and serve immediately.

Nutritional Information (per serving):

- Calories: 220
- Protein: 10g
- Fat: 1.5g
- Carbohydrates: 45g
- Fiber: 4g
- Sugar: 30g

Berry Blast Collagen Smoothie

Prep Time: 5 mins

Total Time: 5 mins

Servings: 2 glasses

Ingredients:

- 1 cup frozen mixed berries
- 1/2 cup ice made with filtered or spring water

- 1 cup almond milk
- 1 scoop collagen powder
- 1/2 banana
- 1 tbsp almond butter
- 1 tsp honey or maple syrup (optional)

Directions:

1. Combine frozen mixed berries, ice, almond milk, collagen powder, banana, and almond butter in a blender.
2. Add honey or maple syrup if desired.
3. Blend until smooth and creamy.
4. Pour into glasses and serve immediately.

Nutritional Information (per serving):

- Calories: 250
- Protein: 12g
- Fat: 10g
- Carbohydrates: 30g
- Fiber: 8g
- Sugar: 16g

Citrus Sunrise Collagen Smoothie

Prep Time: 5 mins

Total Time: 5 mins

Servings: 2 glasses

Ingredients:

- 1 cup orange juice
- 1/2 cup ice made with filtered or spring water
- 1/2 cup Greek yogurt

- 1 scoop collagen powder
- 1 tbsp honey
- 1/2 tsp vanilla extract
- Optional: orange zest for garnish

Directions:

1. In a blender, combine orange juice, ice, Greek yogurt, collagen powder, honey, and vanilla extract.
2. Blend until smooth and creamy.
3. Pour into glasses.
4. Garnish with orange zest if desired.
5. Serve immediately.

Nutritional Information (per serving):

- Calories: 180
- Protein: 8g
- Fat: 1g
- Carbohydrates: 35g
- Fiber: 1g
- Sugar: 25g

Green Goddess Collagen Smoothie

Prep Time: 5 mins

Total Time: 5 mins

Servings: 2 glasses

Ingredients:

- 1 cup spinach
- 1/2 cup cucumber, chopped
- 1/2 cup pineapple chunks

- 1/2 avocado
- 1 cup coconut water
- 1 scoop collagen powder
- Juice of 1 lime
- Optional: mint leaves for garnish

Directions:

1. Blend spinach, cucumber, pineapple chunks, avocado, coconut water, collagen powder, and lime juice until smooth.
2. Pour into glasses.
3. Garnish with mint leaves if desired.
4. Serve immediately.

Nutritional Information (per serving):

- Calories: 200
- Protein: 7g
- Fat: 6g
- Carbohydrates: 30g
- Fiber: 8g
- Sugar: 18g

Vanilla Berry Collagen Smoothie

Prep Time: 5 mins

Total Time: 5 mins

Servings: 2 glasses

Ingredients:

- 1 cup mixed berries (strawberries, raspberries, blueberries)
- 1/2 cup ice made with filtered or spring water
- 1 cup unsweetened almond milk

- 1 scoop collagen powder

- 1/2 tsp vanilla extract

- 1 tbsp honey or maple syrup (optional)

Directions:

1. Combine mixed berries, ice, almond milk, collagen powder, vanilla extract, and honey or maple syrup in a blender.

2. Blend until smooth and creamy.

3. Pour into glasses and serve immediately.

Nutritional Information (per serving):

- Calories: 180

- Protein: 10g

- Fat: 3g

- Carbohydrates: 25g

- Fiber: 5g

- Sugar: 15g

MEAL PLAN

Day 1

- **Breakfast:** Tropical Collagen Smoothie
- **Lunch:** Grilled chicken salad with mixed greens
- **Dinner:** Baked salmon with roasted vegetables

Day 2

- **Breakfast:** Berry Blast Collagen Smoothie
- **Lunch:** Quinoa and roasted vegetable salad
- **Dinner:** Stir-fried tofu with broccoli and brown rice

Day 3

- **Breakfast:** Citrus Sunrise Collagen Smoothie
- **Lunch:** Turkey and avocado wrap with spinach
- **Dinner:** Grilled shrimp skewers with quinoa tabbouleh

Day 4

- **Breakfast:** Green Goddess Collagen Smoothie
- **Lunch:** Lentil soup with a side of whole grain bread
- **Dinner:** Baked chicken breast with steamed asparagus

Day 5

- **Breakfast:** Vanilla Berry Collagen Smoothie
- **Lunch:** Greek salad with grilled chicken
- **Dinner:** Baked sweet potato with black beans and salsa

Day 6

- **Breakfast:** Tropical Collagen Smoothie

- **Lunch:** Veggie stir-fry with tofu and brown rice
- **Dinner:** Grilled steak with roasted Brussels sprouts

Day 7

- **Breakfast:** Berry Blast Collagen Smoothie
- **Lunch:** Quinoa salad with chickpeas, cucumber, and feta cheese
- **Dinner:** Baked cod with lemon and herbs, served with sautéed spinach

Day 8

- **Breakfast:** Citrus Sunrise Collagen Smoothie
- **Lunch:** Turkey and hummus wrap with mixed greens
- **Dinner:** Spaghetti squash with marinara sauce and turkey meatballs

Day 9

- **Breakfast:** Green Goddess Collagen Smoothie
- **Lunch:** Lentil and vegetable curry with brown rice
- **Dinner:** Grilled chicken Caesar salad

Day 10

- **Breakfast:** Vanilla Berry Collagen Smoothie
- **Lunch:** Caprese salad with grilled chicken
- **Dinner:** Baked salmon with quinoa and steamed broccoli

Day 11

- **Breakfast:** Tropical Collagen Smoothie

- **Lunch:** Chickpea salad with mixed greens, tomatoes, and cucumber
- **Dinner:** Turkey chili with avocado slices

Day 12

- **Breakfast:** Berry Blast Collagen Smoothie
- **Lunch:** Veggie sushi rolls with edamame
- **Dinner:** Stir-fried tofu with mixed vegetables and brown rice

Day 13

- **Breakfast:** Citrus Sunrise Collagen Smoothie
- **Lunch:** Greek yogurt parfait with granola and fresh fruit
- **Dinner:** Baked chicken thighs with roasted carrots and potatoes

Day 14

- **Breakfast:** Green Goddess Collagen Smoothie
- **Lunch:** Lentil and vegetable soup with whole grain bread
- **Dinner:** Grilled shrimp with quinoa salad

Day 15

- **Breakfast:** Vanilla Berry Collagen Smoothie
- **Lunch:** Turkey and avocado wrap with spinach
- **Dinner:** Baked sweet potato with black bean chili

Day 16

- **Breakfast:** Tropical Collagen Smoothie
- **Lunch:** Quinoa salad with roasted vegetables and feta cheese
- **Dinner:** Grilled steak with roasted Brussels sprouts

Day 17

- **Breakfast:** Berry Blast Collagen Smoothie
- **Lunch:** Greek salad with grilled chicken
- **Dinner:** Baked cod with lemon and herbs, served with sautéed spinach

Day 18

- **Breakfast:** Citrus Sunrise Collagen Smoothie
- **Lunch:** Turkey and hummus wrap with mixed greens
- **Dinner:** Spaghetti squash with marinara sauce and turkey meatballs

Day 19

- **Breakfast:** Green Goddess Collagen Smoothie
- **Lunch:** Lentil and vegetable curry with brown rice
- **Dinner:** Grilled chicken Caesar salad

Day 20

- **Breakfast:** Vanilla Berry Collagen Smoothie
- **Lunch:** Caprese salad with grilled chicken
- **Dinner:** Baked salmon with quinoa and steamed broccoli

Day 21

- **Breakfast:** Tropical Collagen Smoothie
- **Lunch:** Chickpea salad with mixed greens, tomatoes, and cucumber
- **Dinner:** Turkey chili with avocado slices

CONCLUSION

In conclusion, the discussion thus far has centered around the importance of collagen in maintaining overall health and well-being, as well as various ways to incorporate collagen into one's diet through recipes for smoothies, salads, soups, desserts, and beverages. Collagen, the most abundant protein in the human body, plays a crucial role in maintaining the structure and integrity of our skin, bones, joints, and other connective tissues. As we age, our bodies produce less collagen, leading to signs of aging such as wrinkles, joint pain, and decreased bone density. Therefore, ensuring an adequate intake of collagen through diet becomes increasingly important as we grow older.

The recipes provided offer delicious and nutritious options for incorporating collagen into daily meals and snacks. From refreshing smoothies packed with fruits, greens, and collagen powder to hearty soups and salads filled with collagen-rich ingredients like bone broth, chicken, fish, and leafy greens, there are numerous ways to boost collagen intake while enjoying flavorful and satisfying dishes. Additionally, desserts and beverages infused with collagen offer a sweet and indulgent way to support skin health and promote overall vitality.

By following a collagen-rich diet, individuals can not only improve the appearance of their skin but also support joint health, strengthen bones, and promote overall wellness. Moreover, the recipes presented here are not only beneficial for those looking to enhance their collagen intake but also for anyone seeking to adopt a nutritious and balanced diet. Incorporating a variety of whole foods, including fruits, vegetables, lean proteins, and healthy fats, can provide essential nutrients that support optimal health and vitality.

As we embark on the journey to prioritize our health and well-being, it's important to remember that small changes can lead to significant improvements over time. By making conscious choices to nourish our bodies with nutrient-rich foods like those featured in the recipes provided, we can take proactive steps towards achieving our health goals and living our best lives. As Hippocrates once said, "Let food be thy medicine and medicine be thy food." This timeless quote serves as a reminder of the profound impact that our dietary choices can have on our overall health and serves as a source of motivation to prioritize wellness in our daily lives. So, let's embrace the power of collagen-rich foods and embark on a journey to vibrant health and vitality.